Reviews of *Prevent and Cure* D…

This book could save the NHS!

One person in four (and rising) has metabolic syndrome in this country. It leads to the epidemics of diabetes, heart disease, stroke, Alzheimer's and cancer that are drowning our health services. Fix it and you could save the NHS from drowning. This book shows us how.

In 1958, Dr Richard Mackarness wrote a book called *Eat Fat and Grow Slim*, which pretty much did what it said on the cover*. So more than half a century ago someone figured this out and offered a solution; but then what happened? We as a species spent half a century believing that fats are bad for us and so avoiding them, and all the time getting fatter, sicker, dumber and often deader.

Now that whole mythology is falling apart, and with the help of books like this we can re-learn what we were somehow fooled into forgetting - how to get and stay well, fit and strong with practical nutrition.

Dr Sarah Myhill provides a clear, and often entertaining, explanation of how sugar poisons us, how we become addicts, and how to get out of this 'jail' free. She owns up to having been a sugar-junkie herself (although I must say she hides her addiction well – unless it is to that insane horse-riding stuff she does). So if she says 'It may be hard, but you can do it', you know you can believe her.

You don't need to have diabetes, or even metabolic syndrome, to benefit from this book; it offers a solution to nearly every disease you are likely to encounter in this century and this society. If GPs gave this out to their patients first, before prescribing drugs, we might indeed save the NHS.

Dr Damien Downing MB BS, MRSB President, British Society of Ecological Medicine

Dr Sarah Myhill is a medical pioneer and an explorer, a brave open-minded healer who seeks out that which works and makes people better. Her thousands of patients who have seen the irreversible being reversed under her care are testament to that. In this revelatory book, she turns her attention to the lifestyle disease of our time, and demonstrates that it is very preventable and treatable without drugs. It is a book that demands to be on the shelves of any intelligent, enquiring person.

Bryan Hubbard, *What Doctors Don't Tell You*

* Nearly 20 years later Dr Mackarness wrote *Not All in the Mind*, which introduced Britain to the idea of food allergy and intolerance, and led to the setting up of the British Society for Nutritional Medicine – now it is for Ecological Medicine – of which both Dr Myhill and I are long-term members.

This practical, evidence-based book reviewing mechanisms leading to diabetes, challenges current mainstream thinking about the impact of the modern Western diet on our health. Dr Myhill's passion, curiosity and conclusions are both compelling and motivating. As both a doctor and a patient, I am only too aware that empowering people is the key to optimum health. I can't wait to start making changes to my own diet.

Nina Lawrence, MB BChir, Consultant Psychiatrist

Dr Sarah Myhill's latest book, *Prevent and Cure Diabetes*, is another masterpiece and the reader can soon see why Sarah has such a stellar reputation amongst her many thousands of grateful patients. In Britain, medical progress is skewed by Big Pharma's need to make a profit. An oppressed medical profession often defaults to orthodoxy, custom and practice, established dogma and N.I.C.E. Guidelines - it protects them in an age of complaint and litigation. Research and the essential challenge to dogma and the establishment are sadly, often met with sneering, dismissal or personal attack rather than scientific debate which would either confirm or constructively refine new ideas.

If we fear to challenge, we never improve; we never progress.

Sarah Myhill has the courage and the expansive mind to think the unthinkable from which all progress is made. She lives in the scientific world of 'EDPIE':

Evaluate - Diagnose - Plan - Implement - Evaluate again.

Crucially, this is a permanently recurring process for her in all her books, where her humility and public gratitude to her sources mask her stunning and major contribution and collation of the overall product. Interestingly, many of her earlier ideas, derided at the time, have since slipped, unappreciated, into mainstream acceptance...

This book helps the professional and lay person alike. It gives clear guidance on how both to treat and to prevent disease with tools available to us all. The eloquence makes it hard to put down - a real 'page-turner'. When could we last say that of a medical book?

Nigel Williams BSc MSc CMath MIMA MCMI FRSA, Headmaster

I am a patient of Dr Myhill's. I was diagnosed with diabetes in 2010 since when I have been following her advice as detailed in this book. Annual blood tests have been perfect. I am taking no prescription medication, only nutritional supplements. I am as fit, well and mentally sharp in my 80s as I have ever been and much looking forward to the next 20 years.

Ken Maggs, retired teacher

Prevent and Cure DIABETES

Delicious Diets, Not Dangerous Drugs

Don't Dine with the Devil

Dr Sarah Myhill MB BS
and
Craig Robinson MA (Oxon)

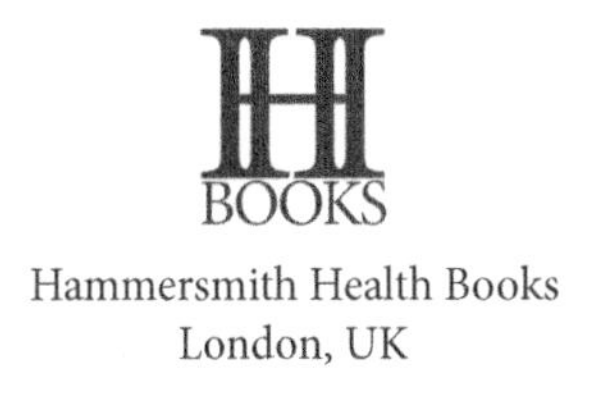

Hammersmith Health Books
London, UK

Dedication

SM: 'To my lovely patients, who have been willing guinea pigs and most forgiving when my suggestions have not worked. However, in doing so, they have pushed forward the frontiers of practical medicine.'

CR: 'To my wife, Penny, without whom I would not be here.'

First published in 2016 by Hammersmith Health Books – an imprint of
Hammersmith Books Limited
14 Greville Street, London EC1N 8SB, UK
www.hammersmithbooks.co.uk

Reprinted 2016, 2018

The information contained in this book is for educational purposes only. It is the result of the study and the experience of the authors. Whilst the information and advice offered are believed to be true and accurate at the time of going to press, neither the authors nor the publisher can accept any legal responsibility or liability for any errors or omissions that may have been made or for any adverse effects which may occur as a result of following the recommendations given herein. Always consult a qualified medical practitioner if you have any concerns regarding your health.

British Library Cataloguing in Publication Data: A CIP record of this book is available from the British Library.

Print ISBN 978-1-78161-077-0
Ebook ISBN 978-1-78161-078-7

Commissioning editor: Georgina Bentliff
Designed and typeset by: Julie Bennett, Bespoke Publishing Ltd
Cover design by: Julie Bennett, Bespoke Publishing Ltd
Index: Dr Laurence Errington
Production: Helen Whitehorn, Path Projects Ltd
Printed and bound by: TJ International Ltd, Padstow, Cornwall, UK.

Contents

About the Authors

Dr Sarah Myhill MB BS qualified in medicine (with Honours) from Middlesex Hospital Medical School in 1981 and has since focused tirelessly on identifying and treating the underlying causes of health problems, especially the 'diseases of civilisation' with which we are beset in the West. She has worked in the NHS and private practice and for 17 years was the Hon. Secretary of the British Society for Ecological Medicine, which focuses on the causes of disease and treating through diet, supplements and avoiding toxic stress. She helps to run, and lectures at, the Society's training courses and also lectures regularly on organophosphate poisoning, the problems of silicone, and chronic fatigue syndrome. Visit her website at www.drmyhill.co.uk

Craig Robinson MA took a first in Mathematics at Oxford University in 1985. He then joined Price Waterhouse and qualified as a Chartered Accountant in 1988, after which he worked as a lecturer in the private sector, and also in the City of London, primarily in Financial Sector Regulation roles. Craig first met Sarah in 2001, as a patient for the treatment of his CFS, and since then they have developed a professional working relationship, where he helps with the maintenance of www.drmyhill.co.uk, the moderating of Dr Myhill's Facebook groups and other ad hoc projects, as well as with the editing and writing of her books.

Authors' roles

Use of the first person singular in this book refers to me, Dr Sarah Myhill. One can assume that the medicine and biochemistry are mine, as edited by Craig Robinson, and that the classical and mathematical references are Craig's.

Craig has been an essential part of this book. As a doctor, I tend to assume much information. Craig is a First Class Oxford mathematician who thinks logically. He has written out the medico-speak and ensured the writing flows in a biologically plausible and comprehensible way. Thank you Craig!

SM

Morning Surgery at Dr Myhill's

MONDAY

FED-UP PATIENT: 'Just not feeling myself, tired, irritable, foggy brain, can't lose weight, can't get fit.'
Dr M: '...and your diet is...?'
QUIZZICAL PATIENT (thinking, 'This is a bit weird; normally at this point other doctors start writing a prescription'): 'Well, I ...er ... I eat a normal, healthy, balanced diet..."
Dr M---: '...So breakfast is ...?'
SMUG PATIENT (giving confident smile thinking that Dr Myhill will be really impressed): 'Cereal or muesli, with low-fat milk and sweetener, orange juice, toast, margarine and marmalade. Tea.'
Dr M (remember that this old matriarch, Dr M, is becoming increasingly grumpy and, in consequence, even more direct): Flashes smug patient a hot stare.
CRUSHED PATIENT (with weakening voice): '...Sandwiches for lunch, fruit for snacks, pasta for supper ...all cooked in sunflower oil, you know!'
Dr M: 'So you have metabolic syndrome. And if you carry on like this you will get diabetes...'
DEFENSIVE PATIENT: '...but I eat my five a day, I've cut out all fat and my cholesterol is good. I have done everything I have been told to...'
Dr M: '...and then you will die prematurely from cancer, heart disease or dementia – no time to explain – read this book!'

TUESDAY

CRESTFALLEN PATIENT: 'I've started the book. And yes, I am a carbohydrate addict.'
Dr M: 'You admit it...and yes...?'
SHEEPISH PATIENT: '...and my diet is abnormal, unhealthy and unbalanced.'
Dr M: 'Keep reading...'

WEDNESDAY

THOUGHTFUL PATIENT: 'Now I understand the "Why"s and "What to do"s..., but the *changes* are so difficult.'
Dr M: 'Keep reading, take a leap of faith and just DO IT.'

THURSDAY

DETERMINED PATIENT (with a steely look in the eye): 'OK, I am going to do it but I will hate you forever.'
Dr M: 'Read the book again!'

FRIDAY

MISERABLE PATIENT: 'I am feeling effing awful!'
Dr M: 'Jolly good – that's really made my day! You have the classic withdrawal reaction symptoms. You will do well. Carry on. Stick with it!'

ONE MONTH LATER

TRIUMPHANT PATIENT: 'I have never felt so well in my life! I have lost a stone in weight. I can go all day. My brain is sharp. I just feel so cheerful. I have horizons and a future.'
Dr M: 'Remember this moment. You will forget. Addicts always do. When you do forget and relapse – read the book again *and* remember this moment!'
CONSPIRATORIAL PATIENT (leaving, with confidential sly glance): '...and the sex is great again...'

Preamble

The word 'diabetes' comes from the Greek meaning 'siphon', illustrating one late-presenting symptom of diabetes – namely, excessive urination and excessive thirst.

There are two main categories of diabetes:

1. Diabetes mellitus (excessive urination caused by sugar in the urine). Here the 'mellitus' is derived from the Latin, meaning honeyed or sweet, and is a reference to the excessive sugar found in urine in this category of diabetes.
2. Diabetes insipidus (excessive urination caused by abnormal pituitary function and therefore kidney function). Here the 'insipidus', deriving again from the Latin, means pale, or tasteless, and refers to the pale urine seen in this category of diabetes.

Further, diabetes mellitus has been split into two types: type 1 and type 2. Both types have to do with the loss of control of blood sugar, but for two different reasons:

Diabetes type 1 is an autoimmune condition which results because the insulin-producing cells of the pancreas have been destroyed. The commonest cause of this is autoimmunity but some other pancreatic diseases will present with type 1 diabetes.

These patients all require insulin by injection because the pancreas cannot produce the amount of insulin they need.

Diabetes type 2 is the loss of control of blood sugar for all reasons other than the loss of insulin-producing cells in the pancreas. This process of losing control starts with what is called 'metabolic syndrome' (page 239) and, given time, inevitably progresses to diabetes. The treatment of both metabolic syndrome and diabetes – namely, to reverse that progression – is the same.

This book is largely about diabetes type 2. However, type 1 diabetes can be greatly improved by all the strategies that are also used to treat type 2 diabetes. If these treatments are put in place, even though insulin will always be needed, blood sugar control will be much improved, and insulin requirements substantially reduced. This, in turn, will reduce the risk of complications. In the not too distant future, type 1 diabetes will be curable with stem cell therapy – roll on that day! Type 2 diabetes can only be cured by restoring evolutionarily correct diets and lifestyles, as detailed in this book.

Chapter 1

Introduction – why this book?

I see many patients with diabetes. It is clear that the conventional advice given to them does not address the causes of their condition and so cannot reverse it or prevent progression. Conventional dietary and medical advice is not just inadequate; by focusing on calorie counting, cutting out fats, eating carbohydrates with every meal, and the taking of prescription drugs, it is also uninspiring and disempowering, and – even worse – it allows the disease to progress. Patients following this advice inexorably move on to more prescription drugs and premature death.

This is because the conventional medical approach fails to address the key issues of carbohydrate addiction (p 29), glycogen sponges (p 225), fermenting guts (p 152), hormonal deficiencies (p 63), the causes of insulin resistance (p 8), how to reverse metabolic inflexibility (p 239) and, also, how to establish keto-adaption (p 66). Without a full understanding of these issues, we have neither the tools, nor the mental, physical and emotional determination, to put into place the necessary lifestyle and dietary changes to reverse metabolic syndrome (p 239) and diabetes.

Already our glorious National Health Service is being overwhelmed by the complications of metabolic syndrome and diabetes. We all have it within our power to reverse this progression. We must wake up to Darwin's 'survival of the fittest' principle. Those people and families who understand the causes of metabolic syndrome and have the determination to reverse it will be the long-term survivors.

Not only must we understand these causes and put into place the changes to reverse the damage that has already been done, but we must *stick* to these changes – these are lifestyle changes for life. Like Darwin's American Monkey,[1] we must learn from the error of our ways:

> *'An American monkey, after getting drunk on brandy, would never touch it again, and thus is much wiser than most men.'*
>
> Charles Darwin (1809–1882)

The ideas which follow are for the most part based on well-researched science. However, for the reader's information, I have indicated where some are less well researched or even speculative. Even so, all are at least biologically plausible and all come with a sound clinical basis from my practice. In addition, all of these ideas pass the 'Do No Harm' test.

As Linus Pauling famously said, to have good ideas we need to have lots of ideas and then throw away the bad ones.[2] It may be that some of what follows will have to be discarded, but, at least no harm will have been done, and I hope that there are enough good ideas here both to enthuse each and every reader and to motivate you all to carry on through with this difficult evolution of individual discovery.

At the very least, there should be enough in this book to make you think.

> *'I cannot teach anybody anything; I can only make them think.'*
> *'Education is the kindling of a flame, not the filling of a vessel.'*
>
> Socrates, Greek philosopher (470/469–399 BC)

Chapter 2

Sugar – our non-essential and dangerous fuel

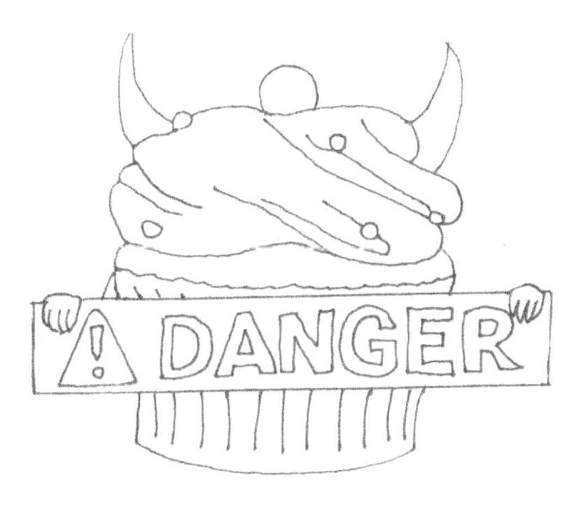

For most of us, sugar in the blood is as essential, but also as dangerous, as petrol in our cars. In my clinical practice I spend more time talking about how the body controls blood sugar than all other subjects put together. I came into this subject through my interest in treating patients with chronic fatigue syndrome: blood sugar levels running too high or too low both result in the symptom of fatigue. Indeed, for many, blood sugar levels running too low can result in unconsciousness and death. (See Chapter 6, page 56 for more on this.) Importantly, this problem of low blood sugar is only a problem in people who fuel their body with carbohydrates and who have developing, or established, metabolic syndrome and metabolic inflexibility. The symptoms of hypoglycaemia (blood sugar that is too low) arise because they cannot switch into the alternative way of fuelling the body – burning fat. Interestingly, once this facility to burn fat has been re-established (called keto-adaptation – see p 66) one becomes much more tolerant of hypoglycaemia simply because the body can happily function on fat in the form of ketone bodies. If the body is happy running on ketones then adrenaline (known as epinephrine in the US) is not poured out – and it is adrenaline that gives us the symptoms of hypoglycaemia. Indeed, Dr Heinz Reinwald reported at a BSEM (British Society of Ecological Medicine) conference how some people can run blood sugars below 1 millimole per litre (mmol/l – conventional [NICE and NHS in the UK] 'normal' is 4 to 5.9 mmol/l before meals and 7.8 90 minutes after)* and not suffer any malign effects. I know this to be the case – sometimes I send off routine blood samples and the report comes back with the blood sugar 'below measurable' – but the patient was completely well at the time of testing.

Over time it has become increasingly apparent to me that this loss of control of blood sugar is driving our modern epidemics of cancer, heart disease and dementia.

Historical note: It was not always so. Maimonides (12th–13th century AD), writing in *Medical Aphorisms*, comments on 'diabetes', in Chapter 8, saying that Galen states that this condition expresses itself through a very heavy thirst and frequent urination but that it is extremely rare in the 'West' and that neither Galen, nor his teachers, had personally come across any cases. He further notes that cases had been reported from Egypt, positing that the cause may be the propensity of the Egyptians, at that time, to take sweet drinks. How right he

* Note: The 'normal' levels given by NICE in the UK are based on a 'normal' population, but we no longer have such as we no longer eat an evolutionarily correct diet. The NICE normal levels are set high, and those for type 2 diabetics are set even higher (4 to 7 before meals and 8.5 90 minutes after) though they should be exactly the same.

may have been in his deductions. Maimonides was an extraordinary person, who prefaced his work on Ethics with the advice: '...one should accept the truth from whatever source it proceeds.'

Sugar is essential in the bloodstream but it is not essential as a food. For millions of years, Man evolved with very low-carbohydrate and sugar diets. He was fuelled by fat, protein and vegetable fibre. Indeed, Dr Heinz Reinwald[3] recognises three ages of nutrition:

1. The Stone Age, of over 2.5 million years finishing about 10,000 years ago, when the diet was ultra-low carbohydrate and largely ketogenic.
2. The Glucogenic Age from 10,000 BC to about 1850, when increasingly humans were fuelled by starches from the Agrarian Revolution.
3. The Glucotoxic Age from 1850 to date, when the Industrial Revolution allowed wholesale access to cheap addictive sugars and refined carbohydrates.

Sugar toxicity problems really came to a head in the 1960s with the great debate[4, 5, 6] spearheaded on the fat side by Dr John Yudkin, Founding Professor of the Department of Nutrition at Queen Elizabeth College London, and on the sugar side by Dr Ancel Keys, American scientist. Keys was backed by the agrochemical industry, the food industry, the pharmaceutical industry, the US Army and the US Government. In such debates, the science is discarded – power and money always trump truth. The Glucotoxic Age took off, consumption of sugar and refined carbohydrates increased exponentially and epidemics of metabolic syndrome and diabetes ensued.

Indeed, it is predicted by some that by the year 2030, up to 50% of some Western populations will have metabolic syndrome and diabetes. My estimate is that over 95% of the current Western population, young and old, already have prodromal (latent) metabolic syndrome – namely, carbohydrate addiction. This epidemic is a direct result of our modern Western diets and lifestyles, these being diets and lifestyles not experienced or practised by our 12th and 13th century forebears. To understand how to prevent, how to diagnose and, of course, how to treat diabetes we must first understand the mechanisms that are driving this epidemic. Attention to these 'driving mechanisms', applied at any stage of either metabolic syndrome or diabetes, will result in prevention, remission and cure. With that, additionally, comes protection against cancer, heart disease and dementia.

Historical note: Herodotus tells of the difference in longevity of the Persians and Ethiopians. He writes of how the Persians ate bread from grain fertilised with dung and that some lived to an age of 80, whilst the Ethiopians, who lived on boiled meat, regularly lived to 120, and that they (the Ethiopians) attributed the 'low' life expectancy of the Persians to the fact that they ate shit! How right the Ethiopians were. *Herodotus, Histories*, circa 440 BC, and as recently reported in Finch 2009.[7]

What is diabetes type 2?

Diabetes type 2 is the end result of years of metabolic havoc as the body progressively loses control of levels of sugar in the blood. The early phase of this metabolic havoc is called 'metabolic syndrome'.

Sugar in the blood is like the petrol in our cars. It is absolutely essential for the human body to work, just as petrol is essential for the engines of our cars to work. However, sugar *in the diet* is not essential except for the non-keto-adapted. There is an important, yet subtle, distinction here that will become clearer as the biochemistry is discussed in more detail; in short – sugar is essential in the blood but is neither essential nor, indeed, at all desirable, in our diets.

If blood sugar levels fall too low, we fall unconscious and become easy prey for a sabre-toothed tiger – or its modern-day equivalent!

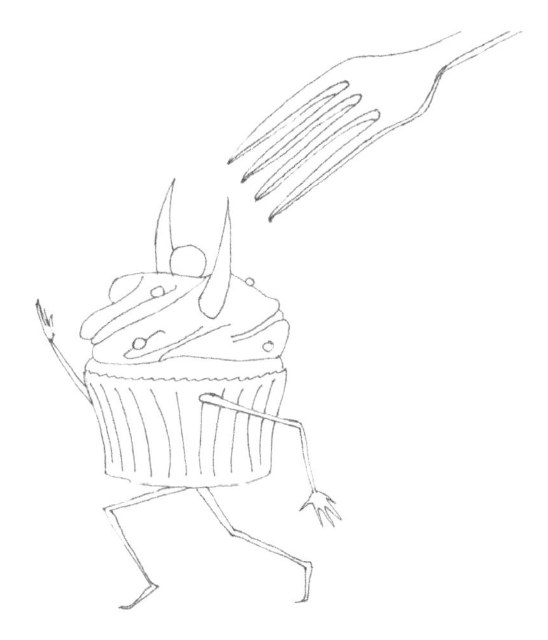

Nature cannot allow the body to run out of fuel, so when things go wrong it errs on the safe side – if we start to lose control of blood sugar, and we cannot correct this by switching into burning fat as an alternative source of energy, then it is preferable to allow blood sugar to run on the high side – short-term gain but long-term pain because, as you will see, high levels of sugar in the blood are horribly damaging to the body. Interestingly, a similar scenario arises in pregnancy – the growing baby is exquisitely sensitive to fuel delivery mechanisms and if sugar levels fall in maternal blood, serious damage to the baby results. So Nature ensures that the mother runs her blood sugars higher than normal to protect the baby. If she has already started to lose control of her blood sugar, then pregnancy may tip her over into frank diabetes (so-called 'gestational diabetes'). What this tells us is that high levels of female sex hormones, as experienced during pregnancy, allow women to run higher blood sugars and this explains why the Pill and HRT (hormone replacement therapy) are both risk factors for metabolic syndrome and diabetes.

Loss of control of blood sugar levels is the first step towards diabetes and is, as stated earlier, called metabolic syndrome. It is also known as 'syndrome X', 'cardiometabolic syndrome', 'insulin resistance syndrome', 'Reaven's syndrome' and 'CHAOS' (Coronary artery disease, Hypertension, Atherosclerosis, Obesity, and Stroke). These are dreadful names designed to confuse patients and make doctors seem clever; doctors love to use difficult, often foreign, words to describe disease and pathology but in doing so obfuscate the underlying causes.

> The preferred language of deception of the medical profession is Latin. Craig studied Latin and remembers the little ditty often murmured by his schoolmates at the beginning of Latin lessons: 'Latin is a language, as dead as it can be; it killed the Ancient Romans, and now it's [insert expletive] killing me.'

The real joke is that most doctors do not know what metabolic syndrome is. Again, let's briefly turn to the wisdom of Maimonides, who states that:

> *'There is one [disease] which is widespread, ... I refer to this: that ... person thinks his mind ... more clever and more learned than it is ... They ... express themselves [not only] upon the science with which they are familiar, but upon other sciences about which they know nothing ... If met with applause ... so does the "disease" itself become aggravated.'*

So, for example, having diagnosed metabolic syndrome in one of my patients, his GP referred him to the renal unit for the treatment of his 'metabolic syndrome', clearly showing his complete misunderstanding of the term. Indeed, a perusal of the obituaries in the *British Medical Journal* (where the cause of death is additionally given) shows that most doctors die from the end result of metabolic syndrome – they too have not understood!

In the 1990s, the *British Medical Journal* made attempts to encourage self-penned obituaries – to be published *post mortem*. The idea was that this would lead to more interesting obituaries, with doctors having more insight into their own deficiencies and failures. It seems that this was a doomed, yet worthy, objective – such insight is clearly missing.

'Any intelligent fool can make things bigger, more complex, and more violent. It takes a touch of genius – and a lot of courage – to move in the opposite direction.'

Internet Meme wrongly attributed to Albert Einstein*

I hope that what follows explains the problems of sugar, the mechanisms by which these problems arise and, most importantly, what must be done to correct the dangers arising from these problems. This will, I hope, provide the intellectual imperative to make the difficult but necessary changes before disease results.

*Note: During the course of obtaining permission to use quotations, Craig contacted the relevant copyrightholders, and for Einstein, this was, for the most part, The Hebrew University of Jerusalem, who kindly replied, stating that, along with virtually every other quote on the Internet attributed to Einstein, the four such quotes contained in this book were wrongly attributed. This is another reminder that one should question everything and not blindly believe all that one reads, or indeed just accept Received Wisdom. In part, this is what this book is about – questioning the accepted practice of the prevention and treatment of diabetes. It is also interesting to note that, in order to give their quotations more gravitas, the Internet Meme'ers added Einstein as originator. This is a common practice also, whereby credence is hoped to be given to an argument or point of view by attaching to it the name of a well-accepted Establishment figure. Again, this tactic has been employed in Established Medicine for centuries.

'There is an old saying that things don't [just] happen; they are made to happen.'

John F Kennedy* (1917–1963)

*We are very grateful to The Textual Archives of the John F Kennedy Presidential Library for helping with this quotation which can be accessed here: http://www.presidency.ucsb.edu/ws/?pid=9430 and, indeed, listened to here: http://www.jfklibrary.org/Asset-Viewer/Archives/JFKWHA-223-001.aspx This quotation was made by John F Kennedy in his Address at the University of North Dakota, 25 September 1963, and is in the Public Domain.

Chapter 3

How sugar damages the body – mechanisms, symptoms and disease

Sugar is extremely damaging to the body for many reasons. It is damaging to the body in high levels, it is damaging to the body in low levels, and the swinging of levels between the two is additionally damaging because of the hormonal response to those rapid changes. I call this the blood-sugar rollercoaster – it is often described as a 'hypoglycaemic tendency' ('hypo' meaning 'below', from the Greek) – but it is the whole rollercoaster that causes metabolic havoc – not just the dips.

If we constantly eat carbohydrate foods, this is a rollercoaster which just keeps on going, and along with the metabolic havoc, there are associated mood swings which mirror the ride. These emotions are very similar to those documented by Barry Ritholtz, in his financial writings on the rollercoaster ride experienced by investors in risky stocks (see Figure 1 from www.ritholtz.com/blog/).[8] People who are regularly feeling these emotions, and in particular are experiencing them cyclically, are most likely already on the blood-sugar rollercoaster:

Returning to the medical case in point, in metabolic syndrome and diabetes any or all of the following problems can result. In each case, a description of the problem is followed by symptoms and diseases that may result from that problem, thereby giving clues as to whether this may be an issue in a particular individual.

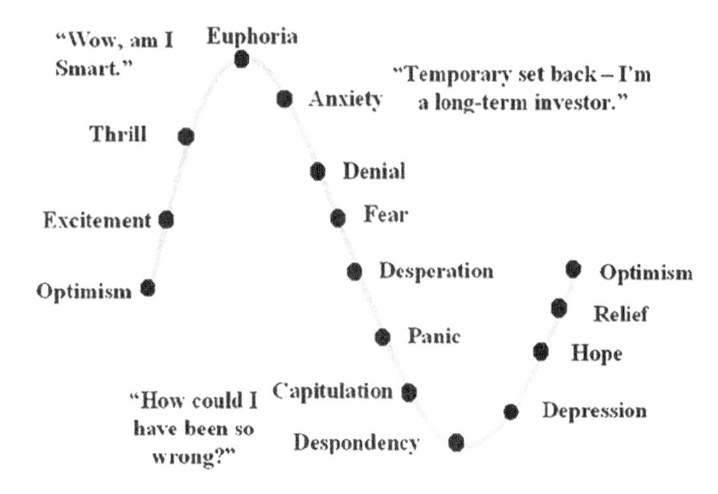

Figure 1: *The financial rollercoaster ride (with permission from Barry Ritholtz)*

A – Sugar is damaging to the body at high levels

1. Sugar is sticky

Sugar is sticky stuff; it sticks onto and damages anything and everything. These sticky conglomerates are called 'advanced glycation end products' (see page 212) – the acronym is AGEs. Indeed, one way to measure our loss of control of blood sugar is to measure sugar stuck onto haemoglobin – 'glycosylated haemoglobin' (HbA1c).

As sugar can stick onto anything, high blood sugar will:

a) Accelerate the normal ageing process (see page 25 for more on this).

b) Stick to proteins and possibly denature them (irreparably change their structure) in such a way as to cause prion disorders, such as Alzheimer's disease. Indeed, Alzheimer's has been renamed type 3 diabetes. In a detailed review – 'Alzheimer's Disease Is Type 3 Diabetes – Evidence Reviewed' the authors Monte and Wands (2008) concluded that: 'Altogether, the results from

Table 1: *Problems with sugar because it is sticky*

Symptoms of high blood sugar	Diseases of high blood sugar
Look ugly*. (Indeed, beauty is how we choose our sexual partners – we also call it attractiveness.) Look old before our time. Cellulite. Note: Being beautiful* reflects inner good health and therefore the ability to procreate. Historically, being fat was deemed beautiful since modest fat meant fertility. Indeed, attractiveness is also determined by breast size (in females) which reflects a mother's potential ability to feed her newborn baby. Attractiveness is also judged by kissing ability, which reflects the mother's ability to wean her baby as she chews food and reduces it to a manageable morsel before kissing it into the infant's mouth. (Male beauty is measured in other ways!) I use the terms 'ugly' and 'beautiful' here in the evolutionary sense of attractiveness – that is, the desirable attributes of a sexual partner for the purposes of procreation. The selfish gene theories of Richard Dawkins (*The Selfish Gene*, 1976)[10] tell us that the only function of life is to procreate. This is a world apart from the 'feminine beauty ideal', a notion that physical attractiveness is one of a woman's most important assets, and something that all women should strive to achieve and maintain.	**Arteriosclerosis** leading to heart disease, stroke, gangrene, retinopathy, micro-angiopathy. (Low levels of friendly HDL cholesterol are an indicator as this is used up in the business of healing and repairing sugar and blood pressure damage to arteries.) Arteriosclerosis combined with prions causes the symptoms of dementia. **Prion disorders**, such as Alzheimer's. **Non-alcoholic fatty liver disease.** **Eye disease** – cataracts, macular degeneration and glaucoma. **Sticky blood and platelets** – venous thrombosis, deep vein thrombosis (DVT) and pulmonary embolus. **Neuropathy** – loss of sensation in the hands and feet (a typical result of diabetes). **Nephropathy** – damage to the kidney (as a result, protein (albumin) leaks into the urine). **Erectile dysfunction** in men (damage to arteries and to nerves) and low testosterone. Possibly, **age-related hearing loss.**

these studies provide strong evidence in support of the hypothesis that AD represents a form of diabetes mellitus that selectively afflicts the brain.'[9] Other prion disorders include Parkinson's and motor neurone disease.

c) Stick to the lining of arteries and damage them directly. The healing and repair process is called arteriosclerosis and the scar tissue that results stiffens and narrows the arteries. A recent arteriosclerotic 'plaque' or scab can break off to cause strokes and infarctions (blockages).

d) Stick to fats, causing lipodystrophy (see page 236). Under the skin this may result in an irregular loss of fat manifesting as cellulite. Loss of fat from the face causes the haggard appearance of premature ageing.

e) Stick to nerves and damage them.

2. Sugar is a growth promoter

Sugar is a growth and, therefore, cancer promoter. What distinguishes cancer cells from normal human cells is how they get their energy. Healthy human cells should be fuelled by ketones from fat and short-chain fatty acids (SCFAs) from the fermentation of vegetable fibre in the large bowel. By contrast, cancer cells can only be fuelled by sugar. Normally, cells in the body are powered by mitochondria. These engines, contained within and delivering energy to all living cells, achieve such by burning acetate (from ketones, SCFAs, sugars or protein) in the presence of oxygen. This is called aerobic metabolism. By contrast, cancer cells switch off their mitochondria – indeed this may be part of the mechanism by which they become cancerous because it is mitochondria which control cell suicide (known as 'apoptosis'). Cancer cells get their energy only through the fermentation of sugar. This is called anaerobic metabolism.

The business of producing cancer requires two clear steps. Firstly, the normal cell has to be damaged in some way and typically this can occur because of ionising radiation, or some sort of carcinogen such as a toxic metal or chemical which damages DNA so as to switch on uncontrolled cell division. The second phase of carcinogenesis has to do with growth promotion – so, for example, we know that growth promoting hormones, such as oestrogen and progesterone, accelerate the growth of sex-hormone sensitive cancers. But the biggest and most unrecognised growth promoter of all is sugar – if you feed these cancers a high-sugar diet, then you will encourage their growth. Indeed, the British Society for Integrative Oncology recommends the ketogenic diet for the treatment of all cancers. Furthermore, some oncologists offer insulin-potentiated chemotherapy. The idea here is that blood sugar levels are lowered by the use of insulin by injection immediately prior to the infusion of chemotherapeutic drugs. Clearly this must be very carefully monitored in hospital. The very low blood sugar level that results renders cancer cells so much more susceptible to the effects of chemotherapy that the total dose of drug used can be substantially reduced – perhaps to as little as 10% of the usual.

Cancer has, indeed, been described as a metabolic disease – fermentation is the 'bio-energetic signature' of cancer cells.* This was first suggested in 1885 by Ernst Freund and confirmed biochemically by Otto Warburg. Warburg won the Nobel Prize in Physiology in 1931 for this work. Cancers are hungry for sugar – so much so that a commonly performed test for cancer is to use a radioactive-labelled sugar and follow its progress through the body with a scan; nearly all of this sugar ends up in the tumour.

Note: Unlike normal cells, which rely upon a process called oxidative phosphorylation – that is to say, energy being released by the oxidation of nutrients – cancer cells rely on fermentation reactions using non-oxidative substrate-level phosphorylation (that is, without oxygen) for their ATP synthesis. Cancer cells can grow in hypoxia (absence of oxygen) as long as they have access to fermentable fuel, such as glucose and glutamine. In brief, normal cells respire using oxygen; cancer cells ferment in the absence of oxygen. I suspect this explains why primary cancer of the heart is so rare – the heart is the best oxygenated organ in the body.

***Table 2:** Problems with sugar – sugar is a growth promoter*

Symptoms of growth promotion	Diseases of growth promotion
Tendency to grow lumps, bumps and cysts (e.g. breast and ovarian). Prostate enlargement. Tallness and fatness – being tall and fat are both known risk factors for cancer.	Polycystic ovarian syndrome. All cancers. Benign growths.

When I talk about blood sugar levels, I mean those in the systemic (whole body) circulation. After a carbohydrate meal, sugar pours into the veins immediately around the gut; the blood from these veins is funnelled, via the portal vein, directly to the liver. Blood sugar levels in the portal vein will fluctuate wildly, but the potential for damage is minimal because it is a low-pressure vessel. However, I suspect this constant spiking of sugar levels in the liver explains why cancer so often seeds and grows there.

3. Sugar is pro-inflammatory

The sugar 'petrol' of our engines is extremely dangerous stuff – too much and it bursts into flames. In the body we call this inflammation. Westerners are now suffering from many diseases associated with this pro-inflammatory tendency. We know (see page 180) our modern epidemics of allergy and auto-immunity are being driven by sugar.

Table 3: *Problems with sugar – sugar is pro-inflammatory*

Symptoms of inflammation	Diseases of inflammation
Itch, pain, rash, fever, redness, swelling, fluid retention, diarrhoea, vomiting and others. Inflammatory markers in the blood tend to be high – e.g. C-reactive protein, ESR (see page 40), plasma viscosity. (Note that a normal result does not mean no allergy or inflammation.)	Allergy – asthma, eczema, urticaria, hay fever, osteo-arthritis, irritable bowel, inflammatory bowel disease, migraine, some forms of epilepsy, mouth ulcers and others. Auto-immunity – hypothyroidism and hyperthyroidism, pernicious anaemia, rheumatoid arthritis, scleroderma, nephritis, primary biliary cirrhosis, type 1 diabetes and others. Gout (probably related to fructose).

B – Sugar is damaging if blood levels fall low

If blood sugar levels fall low, and we are unable to correct this because of metabolic inflexibility, we become acutely confused, fall unconscious and die. Because this is so dangerous in the short term, the body has many mechanisms in place to prevent it from falling unconscious and dying. So, thankfully in practice this never happens, except when diabetes is over-treated with drugs or insulin (although my patients tell me that when they experience a 'hypo' – excessively low blood sugar level – they feel as if they are dying!).

Table 4: *Problems with sugar – hypoglycaemia*

Symptoms of low blood sugar	Diseases of low blood sugar
Foggy brain. Poor memory. Inability to concentrate and multitask. Acute confusion, appear 'drunk'. Acute fatigue.	Unconsciousness and death.

C – The blood-sugar rollercoaster

The blood-sugar rollercoaster, as I explained earlier, is my name for the process of rapidly rising levels of blood sugar prompting a release of insulin and the 'happy' brain neurotransmitters followed by rapidly falling levels of blood sugar causing a release of adrenaline. This combined effect switches on addiction.

Wobbly blood sugar levels are highly damaging because of their hormonal effects. These hormonal effects I suspect relate to the *rate* at which levels of sugar rise and fall in the bloodstream. As we lose control of our blood sugar, then eating a high-carbohydrate snack or meal will cause blood sugar levels to spike, and as blood sugar levels make this rapid rise there is an outpouring of insulin in order to protect the body from this dangerous (but addictive) sugar spike. Insulin brings the blood sugar level down by shunting it into fat. However, if this occurs quickly, then blood sugar levels fall precipitously and that results in an outpouring of adrenaline. Adrenaline is responsible for all the symptoms that we call 'hypoglycaemia'.

Hypoglycaemia comes from the Greek words 'hypo' meaning low, 'gly' meaning sugar and 'aemia' meaning blood, and hence has a literal meaning of 'low sugar blood'.

However, the term hypoglycaemia I suspect is a misnomer that relates to at least two issues. Firstly, adrenaline is released in response to poor fuel delivery (lack of sugar and/or ketones in the bloodstream). This means that, in the keto-adapted, the adrenaline symptoms do not arise because these people can switch into fat-burning mode. Secondly, in those who cannot make this switch, it is not just the *absolute* level of blood sugar that causes the symptoms but also the *rate* of change; this means that often people who complain of hypoglycaemia will be told their blood sugar level is normal from a 'snapshot' blood-sugar test result. What they need is a 'video' of their blood sugar level changing over time to make the diagnosis.

Consequences of the rollercoaster spikes in insulin and adrenaline include the following:

a) **High levels of insulin** put us into a metabolic state of laying down fat, and prevent fat burning – this is the major problem of metabolic inflexibility. It is almost impossible to lose weight when insulin levels are high. Furthermore this effect can be sustained for hours.

b) **High levels of adrenaline** make us anxious, irritable and sleepless. This adrenaline release is a major cause of high blood pressure. Indeed, it astonishes me that doctors appear completely unaware of this link so that hypertension is described as 'essential' (of unknown cause) or 'idiopathic' (again, of unknown cause). They may accurately describe it as due to 'stress', but fail to realise the cause of this stress is actually nutritional stress due to loss of control of blood sugar levels.

Sugar has immediate effects on the brain, by various mechanisms, and this is partly responsible for why sugar is so addictive. For people who have lost control of their blood sugar, in the very short term, a carbohydrate rush, or 'hit', will have a calming effect which allows them to concentrate. Inspector Morse used the carbohydrate hit of a pint of beer to solve his murder mysteries – but ended up diabetic and died prematurely. Falstaff too found that alcohol had an inspirational effect.

> *'It ascends me into the brain, dries me there all the foolish and dull and crudy vapours which environ it, makes it apprehensive, quick, forgetive, full of nimble, fiery, and delectable shapes, which delivered o'er to the voice, the tongue, which is the birth, becomes excellent wit.'*
>
> Act IV scene iii of *Henry IV, Part 2* William Shakespeare (1564–1616)

Any parent will report how their child's behaviour changes abruptly with a sugar hit and, much more noticeably, when blood sugar dives and they become irritable and moody. My daughters were often tired and irritable when they came in from school – it was not until supper that their normal good humour and energy were restored.

Table 5: *Problems with sugar – hyperglycaemia*

Symptoms of blood sugar rising rapidly (due to the sugar hit and insulin)	**Diseases of blood sugar rising rapidly** (due to the sugar hit and insulin)
Brain function improves – better concentration, feel calm, relief from depression. Satiety. Triglycerides in the blood are high as insulin shunts excessive sugar into fat.	Obesity and Inability to lose weight. (It is important to recognise that obesity is not the **cause** of diabetes but may be a symptom of metabolic syndrome – indeed, many people with normal weight have metabolic syndrome and diabetes.)

Table 6: *Problems with sugar – the rollercoaster*

Symptoms of blood sugar falling rapidly (due to adrenaline release)	**Diseases of blood sugar falling rapidly** (due to adrenaline release)
Acute anxiety and low mood. Panic attacks. Insomnia. Shaking. Palpitations. Fearfulness. Hunger and intense desire to eat. Weakness. High blood pressure.	Chronic high blood pressure. Premenstrual tension. Chronic anxiety. Depression. Eating disorders (anorexia and bulimia). Obsessive compulsive disorders. Increased tendency to addiction – caffeine, chocolate, nicotine, cannabis, 'social highs', gambling, sexual perversions, exercise.

You will again see the similarities between the mood changes here and those noted by Barry Ritholtz in his financial writings on the rollercoaster ride experienced by investors in risky stocks (see page 12).

D – High *and* low levels of blood sugar impair energy delivery mechanisms and cause fatigue

Sugar can have a direct and profound effect on energy delivery mechanisms. Just as a car needs a fuel supply that is directly linked to demand, so the body needs to provide a fuel source to mitochondria which exactly matches demand. Too much petrol swamping the engine will choke it; too little petrol will starve it. Blood sugar running too high and too low both result in the symptom of fatigue. If energy delivery is impaired in the short term, this results in acute fatigue, and in the long term, chronic fatigue and an acceleration of the normal ageing process. Again it astonishes me that doctors are unaware of this link and that many of their TATT (tired all the time) patients have this problem as a result of this loss of control of blood sugar. The Porter in *Macbeth* recognised the effects of swinging blood sugar on energy delivery mechanisms, as exemplified by alcohol:

> **Macduff**: *What three things does drink especially provoke?*
> **Porter**: *Marry, sir, nose-painting, sleep, and urine. Lechery, sir, it provokes, and unprovokes; it provokes the desire, but it takes away the performance: therefore, much drink may be said to be an equivocator with lechery: it makes him, and it mars him; it sets him on, and it takes him off; it persuades him, and disheartens him; makes him stand to, and not stand to; in conclusion, equivocates him in a sleep, and, giving him the lie, leaves him.*
>
> Act II scene iii *Macbeth* William Shakespeare (1564–1616)

Furthermore, wobbly blood sugar levels impair energy delivery to the immune system and so it reacts inappropriately – healing and repair are impaired, cancer surveillance is impaired, ability to deal with infection is impaired.

E – Sugar encourages infections

Microbes love to ferment sugar. Life is an arms race – you and I are a free lunch for microbes to move in and make themselves at home in our comfortably warm, moist and nourishing bodies (see Appendix 7 , page 157).

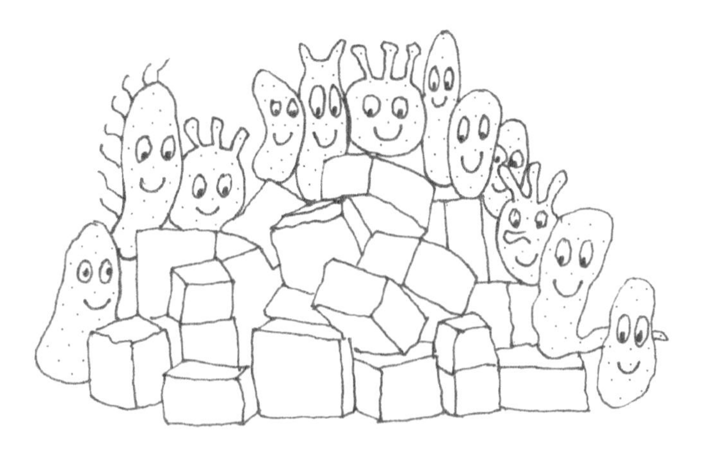

Indeed, our gut is already teeming with microbes, but over thousands of years of evolution we have come to live symbiotically (mutually supportively) with the least harmful of them. However, provide sugar and the harmful flourish. High-sugar diets feed microbes in the mouth (tooth and gum decay – see page 149). Diabetes is often diagnosed when recurrent fungal infections or staphylococcal skin infections start. High-sugar diets give us fermenting mouths (see page 149), fermenting guts (see page 152), fermenting skin (see page 156), fermenting cancers and (I suspect) fermenting brains.

Table 7: *Sugar encourages infection*

Symptoms of infection	Diseases from infection
Teeth feel fuzzy due to dental plaque. Coated tongue – again due to colonies of bacteria or yeast. Gum recession. Need for dental work, including fillings, extraction and root canal work. Recurrent coughs and colds. Tendency to skin infections.	All infectious disease – ear, nose and throat infections, bronchitis and pneumonia, cystitis, acne, cellulitis, infected eczema, boils, meningitis, septicaemia, wound infections, post-operative infections and others. Fungal toenails, thrush, athlete's foot. All viral infections – ear, nose and throat, viral gastroenteritis, influenza, and many others – I suspect sugar puts one at greater risk of all.

F – Sugar in the diet can be fermented in the gut

It is normal and desirable for friendly microbes to ferment fibre in the large bowel, but the stomach and smaller intestine (together, the upper gut) should be relatively microbe-free and the site of digestion, not fermentation. However, high-sugar diets feed unfriendly microbes in the upper gut (fermenting gut – see Appendix 5, page 152, for more detailed information on this). When microbes ferment sugar they produce toxins, such as various alcohols (which further destabilise blood sugar), D-lactate, hydrogen sulphide and many others, including bacterial endotoxins (causing endotoxaemia). Endotoxins switch on the immune system directly and are pro-inflammatory. Even whole gut microbes easily spill over into the bloodstream and this is called 'bacterial translocation'. Many studies have shown the existence of bacterial translocation and its adverse effects on health, for example that by O'Boyle et al (1998).[11] In addition, one can develop symptoms due to allergy to these microbes (called molecular mimicry), or possibly allergic reactions to bacterial endotoxins.

Table 8: *Fermenting gut symptoms and related diseases*

Symptoms of the fermenting gut	Disease resulting from the fermenting gut (evidence for and biological plausibility)
Acid reflux. Bloating. Wind. Rumbling gut. Irritable bowel syndrome – diarrhoea and/or constipation. Mucus and blood in stools. Central obesity (being apple shaped) – because fat is dumped where the immune system is busy.	Inflammatory bowel disease (Crohn's and ulcerative colitis). Interstitial cystitis. Ankylosing spondylitis. Rheumatoid arthritis. Polymyalgia rheumatica. Temporal arteritis. Endotoxin disease – septic shock, alcoholic hepatitis, disseminated intravascular coagulation. Switching on of auto-immunity – multiple sclerosis, Guillain–Barré syndrome. Cancer of the mouth, oesophagus, stomach, large bowel and rectum.

G – Sugar in the diet can be fermented in the brain

It is biologically plausible that bacterial translocation into the brain may result in the fermentation of brain neurotransmitters into LSD and amphetamine-like substances. Many psychiatric illnesses, such as manic depression and schizophrenia, could be partly explained by this mechanism. These are not my ideas but those of the Japanese researcher Nishihara.[12] I think of this as fermenting brain.

Table 9: *Fermenting brain – symptoms and related diseases*

Symptoms of the fermenting brain	Diseases of the fermenting brain (evidence for and biological plausibility)
Hyperactivity. Paranoia. Psychopathy. Hallucinations. Out of body experiences.	Depression. Psychosis. Schizophrenia. Manic depression. Bipolar disorder. Autism. Epilepsy and others.

Importantly, the ketogenic diet is highly effective in treating many of these conditions – see later (page 103).

H – Sugar accelerates the normal ageing process

As we age our ability to heal and repair declines. The process of healing and repairing is energy demanding and anything that reduces energy delivery mechanisms will accelerate this. Degenerative conditions occur when our body is damaged faster than the rate at which we can heal and repair. We cannot live, walk, talk and function without tissue damage occurring, but this is healed and repaired during sleep at night. Sugar is damaging to the body for all the reasons listed above. Wobbly blood sugar levels slow the healing and repair process because they impair both sleep and fuel delivery to mitochondria.

It is important to realise that if blood sugar levels are high then this inhibits mitochondrial function, and if blood sugar levels are low then fuel delivery to mitochondria is impaired and so wobbly blood sugars are bad for mitochondria both ways.

Table 10: *Ageing – symptoms and related diseases*

Symptoms of ageing	Diseases of ageing
Look old before our time. Lipodystrophy (loss of fat tissue, e.g. in the face) and so we lose our youthful 'bloom' rapidly.	Degenerative disease and organ failure, such as thinning of skin and hair. Loss of muscle. Loss of bone (osteoporosis). Loss of connective tissue (arthritis). Liver and kidney failure. Heart failure. Brain failure.

In other words, we should be able to avoid the melancholy Jacques's seventh stage of life:

All the world's a stage,
And all the men and women merely players
They have their exits and their entrances,
And one man in his time plays many parts,
His acts being seven ages
……….. Last scene of all,
That ends this strange eventful history,
Is second childishness and mere oblivion,
Sans teeth, sans eyes, sans taste, sans everything.

Act II scene vii *As You Like It* William Shakespeare (1564–1616)

Conclusion

When we are born, a few of us have the genetic potential to live to 120, like the Ethiopians of Herodotus, but few of us actually achieve this. Whilst genetics may be partly to blame, the World Health Organisation states that 90% of disease is environmental. I reckon that most of us have the potential to live to 100. So, perhaps, 90% of us should get to within 90% of the wonderful age of 100, with our faculties largely intact. I guess that life expectancy should be about 90 years – not three, but rather four, score years and 10.

> *'The days of our years are threescore years and ten; and if by reason of strength they be four score years.'*
>
> King James Bible, *Psalm 90:10*
> (I am suggesting another 10!)

Many of the causes of premature death have been successfully addressed by civilisation – these include famine, the cold, infectious disease, accidents and war. We now have a new weapon of mass destruction and that weapon is contained within our supermarkets. Modern diets high in addictive sugars and carbohydrates are now driving our modern epidemics of premature death.

Chapter 4

Diagnosis of diabetes and its precursor, metabolic syndrome

Before getting to the testing stage we can get some very useful clues from a combination of the clinical picture together with commonly done routine tests. However, if you eat what is generally considered a 'normal, healthy, balanced diet' (ho! ho!) based on the intellectually risible food pyramid, then it is likely that you already have carbohydrate addiction and are on the way to metabolic syndrome and diabetes.

In order of priority and ease, the diagnosis can be made from:

- The contents of the supermarket trolley
- Diet
- Snacking
- Tendency to go for other addictions
- Obesity
- The clinical picture

The contents of the supermarket trolley

- Bread, biscuits, cake, pasta, cereals, sugar, waffles, bagels, dough nuts and other such
- Fruit juice, pop, alcohol, "energy" drinks and general junk drinks
- Fruit basket with tropical sweet fruits such as pineapple, melon, bananas, grapes. Apples and pears.

- Sweet dried fruit – sultanas, raisins, dates
- Snack foods – cereal bars, 'energy bars'
- Sweets, toffees, fudges
- Honey, fructose, syrups
- Jams, marmalades, choc spreads
- Artificial sweeteners
- Ice creams and puddings, like cheesecakes and trifle
- Low cocoa-percentage chocolate
- Crisps, corn snacks, popcorn... you get the idea – we call it junk food!

Such a supermarket trolley is very indicative of a diagnosis of carbohydrate addiction, metabolic syndrome and / or diabetes.

> Indeed, I have just returned from a trip to the supermarket. The man in front was placing his purchases at the check-out. I felt myself sighing as the packets of chocolate biscuits, crisps, white bread and sweet drinks piled up. But what moved me to an intense desire to shout out were the final three items – paracetamol, ibuprofen and a box of antacids. He was poisoning himself with the carbs, then symptom-suppressing with the drugs. Addiction had blinded him to the obvious.

Diet

Breakfast gives the game away. This is because no food has been consumed overnight and with carbohydrate addiction, blood sugar levels are low in the morning. The need for a carbohydrate-based breakfast indicates metabolic syndrome – typically with consumption of fruit, fruit juice, sweetened tea or coffee, cereals, toast, bread or croissants. 'Oh, but surely porridge and muesli are OK?' so many cry. Often they are not OK – the only way to really find out is to measure blood sugar levels.

> Even now my daughters can hear me groaning when the adverts on

the telly for breakfast cereals come on. I really cannot stop myself. The *Telegraph* recently reported that, 'Children's breakfast cereals can contain **as much as three teaspoons of sugar** – the equivalent of two and a half chocolate biscuits,' and so there are also 'hidden' dangers.[13]

Snacking

The need for a carbohydrate snack or sweet drink is often triggered by falling blood sugar. Many people comment that when they go on holiday and treat themselves to a fry-up for breakfast, they no longer feel hungry before lunch. Snacking is a disaster – it feeds the fermenting mouth and gut, prevents the glycogen sponges (see page 225) squeezing dry, spikes insulin and prevents fat burning.

Carbohydrates with every meal

The symptom of 'not being satisfied' with meat and vegetables is particularly indicative of carbohydrate addiction, with the need for a sweet pudding to 'hit the spot'.

Tendency to go for other addictions

Also highly indicative of carbohydrate addiction is the tendency to have other addictions … such as alcohol, smoking, coffee, chocolate, prescription drugs (yes – many of these are addictive), and 'legal' and illegal highs.

Obesity

Obesity is *not* the cause of metabolic syndrome and diabetes, but may be a symptom of both. Many type 2 diabetics have metabolic syndrome and normal weight and vice versa – obese people may have no signs of metabolic syndrome. It is the constant sugar spikes in the portal vein, the effect of which eventually spills over into the systemic (whole body) circulation, when the liver is overwhelmed, that characterises metabolic syndrome and diabetes. We cannot measure these spikes because the portal vein is buried deep in the abdomen and links the gut to the liver. Interestingly, it is the fatty liver that results which is highly correlated with metabolic syndrome and diabetes – not the fatty rest of the body. Fat in the liver can be measured with MRI scans, but this is an expensive test not routinely available.

The ability to gain and lose weight is an essential survival ploy for all mammals. Think of the hibernating female brown bear who has to survive months of intense cold, pregnancy and breast feeding with no food intake. She achieves this on autumn fat together with the ability to switch into fat burning. She remains completely healthy throughout.

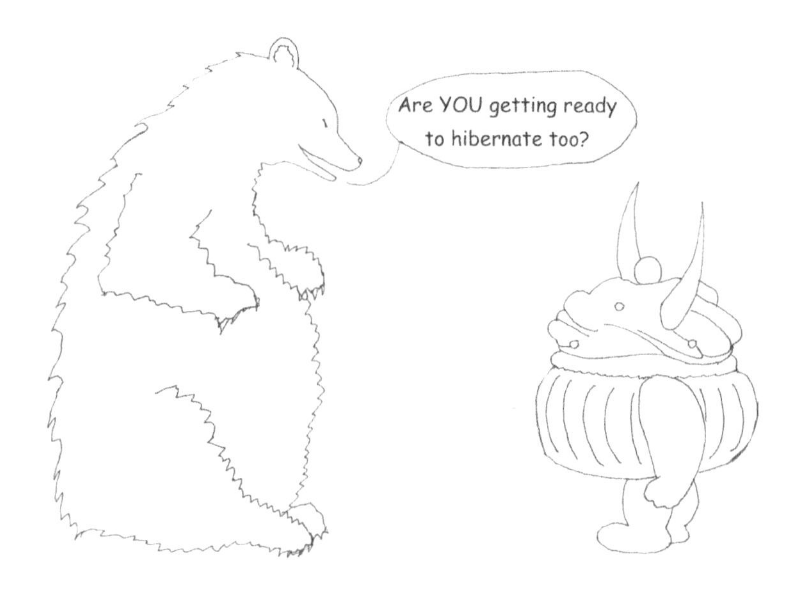

The clinical picture

Table 11: *The signs and symptoms of metabolic syndrome and diabetes*

Symptoms – see above	Diseases — see above
Of high blood sugar. Of low blood sugar. Of growth promotion. Of inflammation. Of the blood-sugar rollercoaster: rapidly rising blood sugar – insulin spike; rapidly falling blood sugar – adrenaline spike. Impaired energy delivery mechanisms. Of infections. Of fermenting gut. Of fermenting brain. Accelerated ageing and degeneration.	Of high blood sugar. Of low blood sugar. Of growth promotion. Of inflammation. Of the blood-sugar rollercoaster. Impaired energy delivery mechanisms. Of infections. Of fermenting gut. Of fermenting brain. Accelerated ageing and degeneration.

> ***Falstaff:*** *You make fat rascals, Mistress Doll.*
> ***Doll Tearsheet:*** *I make them! Gluttony and diseases make them; I make them not.*
>
> Act 2 scene iv *Henry IV Part 2* William Shakespeare

BIOCHEMICAL TESTS FOR METABOLIC SYNDROME AND DIABETES

Metabolic syndrome starts when we lose control of our blood sugar levels. The only true way to test for this therefore is to take the equivalent of a 'video' of such blood sugar levels. This is now possible due to devices that measure blood sugar every few minutes to provide a graph. (These devices are essential in the management of diabetes – page 132.) Indeed, continuous blood sugar monitoring over some time is the only way to truly diagnose metabolic syndrome because this condition results from high blood sugars, low blood sugars and rapidly changing blood sugars. To do otherwise is like trying to see the speed of a car on a stop-start journey from a series of snapshots when what one actually needs is a video recording.

Continuous, or near continuous, blood sugar monitoring

This is the only way to diagnose metabolic syndrome and early diabetes. My view is that all diabetics should routinely use continuous blood sugar monitoring, such as a Dexcom device (see page 132). These devices are currently expensive but many NHS clinics are starting to use them.

In the interim, if one is not convinced by the above clinical picture, then to diagnose metabolic syndrome I suggest very regular blood sugar readings so that a graph can be plotted. There are many cheap devices available to do this, such as Accu-Chek mobile (see page 132). I am a wimp and I would not ask anyone to do anything that I could not do myself. However, the system of obtaining the necessary drop of blood is almost painless. Please do not be put off.

Use Accu-Chek, or equivalent, to measure the following:

a) Fasting blood sugar – that is, after no food for eight hours.
b) Blood sugar immediately after a meal which contains some carbohydrate, then 30 minutes later, one hour later, then every hour for six hours. Include some exercise during this time. This will start to give you an idea of how well you control your blood sugars when your system is stressed by a meal and by exercise.
c) If the result is equivocal, repeat the above by massively stressing the system. Instead of a meal, take a 400 millilitre drink of Lucozade (this contains at least 50 grams of glucose, which represents the NHS standard glucose tolerance test).

During the above trials the blood sugar level should remain between 4.5 and 6.5 mmol/l, with gentle rises and falls between.

The above tests are an excellent way of assessing how well our glycogen sponges (see page 225) are working.

The definition of a 'normal' glucose tolerance test is a one-hour glucose below 10 mmol/l. However, this cannot be a good definition of normal (see page 4). To my mind this already marks a serious deviation from safety – high sugar in the blood is very damaging, and a high level results in spiking insulin and the blood-sugar rollercoaster being triggered. Indeed, we know that one important predictor of longevity has to do with calorie consumption – the less you eat the longer you live. However, I suspect that calories are not the determining factor, but blood sugar – that is, the lower the blood sugar, the less the cumulative damage to the body. In other words, I suspect it is the total area under the curve (blood sugar against time – see Figure 2) that determines longevity. This means by fuelling our bodies with fat and fibre we can minimise that area and extend life expectancy.

We can represent this by constructing stylised graphs of blood sugar against age in years. The blood sugar axis (up the page) is representative only, and without units. Up this axis, we take 0 to be dead and 100 to be very high blood sugar levels. We should be aiming to keep blood sugar levels low. The age axis is simply expressed in years.

In the first graph (Figure 2), we have a person who ran high blood sugar levels all his (or her) life and died aged 60, after having suffered the full range of metabolic syndrome and diabetic complications and symptoms. The shaded area represents a stylised total of blood sugar levels across his entire life and it is this that is the killer of life expectancy. This person got into the habit of running high blood sugars and was never able to kick his addiction. This can be seen from the fact that the shaded area is large – remember, the larger the area, the more the damage that is being done and the shorter the life expectancy, with the full range of awful symptoms associated with metabolic syndrome and diabetes along the way.

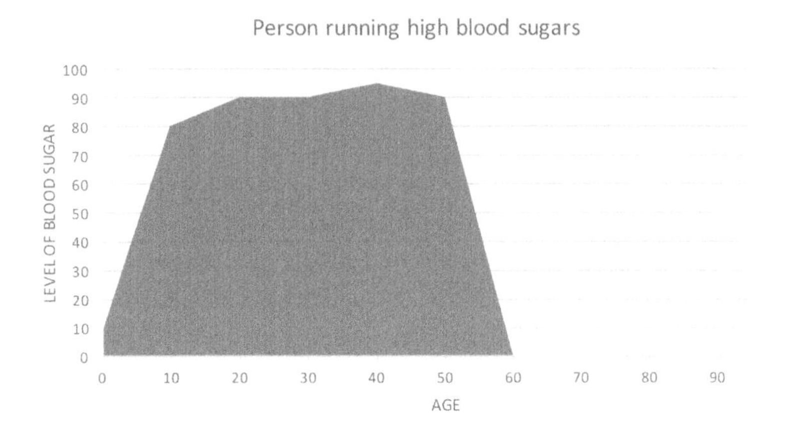

Figure 2: *Profile of blood sugar in a person who has always consumed large amounts of carbohydrate*

In the second graph (Figure 3) we have a person who, initially, ran high levels of blood sugar but then started to learn his (or her) lesson aged somewhere between 10 and 30 years of age. After that time he kept his blood sugar levels low and as a result lived to beyond 100, happily receiving his telegram from the Queen.

In this second case you can see that the shaded area is much smaller than that for the previous person. This means that the damage being done by blood sugar levels is much lower and that this person, who learned his lesson about the dangers of high blood sugars, did not progress along the metabolic syndrome/ diabetes disease pathway but instead reversed this trend, and lived a longer and healthier life.

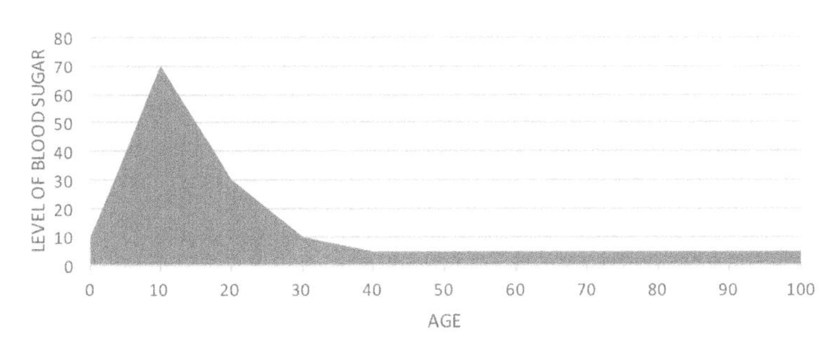

***Figure 3:** Profile of blood sugar in a person who consumed large amounts of carbohydrate in early life but had moved to a ketogenic diet by the age of 40*

In particular, this person learned his lesson early on in life but there is always time – it is never too late to learn (see Chapter 7, page 73). Changing your ways at any stage of life will reverse the progression, and will lead to you feeling healthier and having a longer life expectancy.

Supporting tests may pick up metabolic syndrome or early diabetes, but the diagnosis may be missed

Tests for high blood sugar

Sweet urine – If the blood sugar level spikes, then some will spill over into the urine. Before the days of biochemical tests, high sugar was ascertained by tasting the urine.

> The key to this test, when demonstrating the technique to students, was to dip one finger into the urine, but taste the adjacent finger. Observing students do not notice this sleight of hand and … well, yuck!

Thankfully tasting has been replaced by chemical dipsticks.

Multistix (see page 132) are particularly helpful – not only is glucose detected but also other measures of disease such as blood, protein, white cells, specific gravity and nitrites. The blood sugar has to be very high before glucose starts to spill over and so this is not a good test for diabetes and no test at all for metabolic syndrome.

Glycated haemoglobin (or HbA1c) – This measures sugar stuck on to haemoglobin and so gives an idea of average blood sugars. Sugar is sticky stuff and sticks irreversibly onto haemoglobin in red blood cells. HbA1c reflects average blood sugars over the previous three months. It is used for monitoring blood sugar control in diabetes, but again has been rendered less useful because of changing population reference ranges: some labs state that the normal range is 20 to 40 mmol/mol (4-6% of the total haemoglobin) while for others as high as 53 mmol/mol is deemed acceptable. But it really is a case of the lower the better – every 1 mmol/mol rise in glycated haemoglobin increases diabetic complications by 3%. I would love to see a study measuring levels of glycated haemoglobin in people eating a ketogenic diet. I would predict that the lower the result, the less chance of disease and the greater the chance of a long and healthy life.

'Snap shots' of blood sugar – Even fasting samples, again, are insensitive because they do not show the rate of change of blood sugar levels and may miss a high or a low blood sugar. Often blood sugar has corrected by the time symptoms arise simply because symptoms are due to adrenaline and that results from rapidly falling blood sugars. Adrenaline corrects blood sugar so rapidly that by the time a blood sugar test is done it is often too late.

Serum triglycerides – Insulin shunts glucose into fat and so if blood sugar rises then so do blood levels of triglycerides. This test should be done on a fasting blood sample since there is a normal and temporary rise in triglycerides after eating a fatty meal. This temporary spike of fat levels in the blood is not damaging to blood vessels. High fasting glyceride levels are symptomatic of high insulin due to an overwhelming of the liver's glycogen sponges (see page 225) and sugar spikes in the systemic bloodstream.

Hormonal effects and tests

High insulin – If insulin is high and blood sugar not controlled, then this points to insulin resistance. A fasting insulin level greater than 25 mIU/l suggests insulin resistance.

High adrenaline – We cannot measure blood adrenaline levels easily, but an indirect test of adrenaline is to measure blood pressure. In the short term, high adrenaline levels cause high blood pressure.

Adrenal stress profile – This measures salivary levels of cortisol and DHEA (see cortisol, page 219) over 24 hours. When there is an adrenaline spike this should be followed by a cortisol spike and a DHEA spike. Spiking levels of cortisol in the day reflect a stress response which, most often, is due to falling blood sugar levels. Years of metabolic stress result in adrenal fatigue with low cortisol and DHEA output.

Tests indicating damage to arteries

Low levels of 'friendly' HDL cholesterol – This form of cholesterol is used up in the business of healing and repairing arteries – the higher the result, the better. A level above 20% of the total cholesterol is considered acceptable. I have been collecting HDL total cholesterol percentages in my patients who do high fat, low carb, Stone Age diets. Results are invariably above 30%, usually above 40%, and with a record high of 63% in a particularly fit 93 year old (See Appendix 2, page 139).

Visit your optician – The arteries in the back of the eye can be clearly seen and often early damage is visible there.

Other tests – There are many other tests for arterial disease which are beyond the scope of this book and not routinely or easily available.

Measures of inflammation

These are crude tests for metabolic syndrome but include erythrocyte sedimentation rate, (ESR: <10 mm Hg/hr), C-reactive protein (CRP: <5 mg/l) and plasma viscosity (1.5-1.72 mPa). Again, the normal ranges have risen during my lifetime as a doctor and this reflects our epidemics of metabolic syndrome and the inflammation that accompanies this. These tests are a late indicator of response to damage.

Of course, in practice it is a combination of the clinical picture and test results, together with response to treatment, that gives us the diagnosis. I hate to say it, but the diagnosis of metabolic syndrome is usually obvious. The problem is that carbohydrate addicts are in a constant state of denial and rationalisation of their addiction. This denial and rationalisation is reinforced by the media, advertising and the prevailing 'Received Wisdom'. As it stands, at the moment, the 'personal' evidence for the individual concerned has to be overwhelming before said individual will make the decision to change. It has taken me 34 years of clinical practice and book writing for me to really nail it – I hope your journey is an easier one.

> *'Two things are infinite: the universe and human stupidity; and I'm not sure about the universe.'*
>
> Internet Meme wrongly attributed to Albert Einstein

Note 1: It is unfair to use the word 'stupidity', in its commonly accepted meaning, for patients who do not recognise the full significance of their own symptoms. It is 'cultural denial and rationalisation', reinforced by external factors, that usually lead to this form of 'stupidity'. My patients are among the cleverest people I have met and when presented with the real evidence, they understand the situation very quickly and are highly motivated to make the necessary changes. Often it is those who have not received a formal education who do best because their minds are not clouded by pre-conception and establishment dogma.

Note 2: In 2006, a reclusive Russian mathematician, Grigori Perelman, solved a problem in topology, the Poincaré conjecture, which may eventually help to decide the shape of the universe and thereby questions about its size. Perelman's proof built on work done by Richard Hamilton, an American. In doing so, Perelman was eligible for a Fields Medal (a sort of Nobel Prize for mathematicians), and also for a $1million prize because this problem was one of the so-called Millennium Prizes in mathematics. Perelman declined both the Fields Medal and the $1million prize, stating that 'Everybody understood that if the proof is correct, then no other recognition is needed. I'm not interested in money or fame. I don't want to be on display like an animal in a zoo. I'm not a hero of mathematics. I'm not even that successful; that is why I don't want to have everybody looking at me.'

Sugar– the root of all our addictions

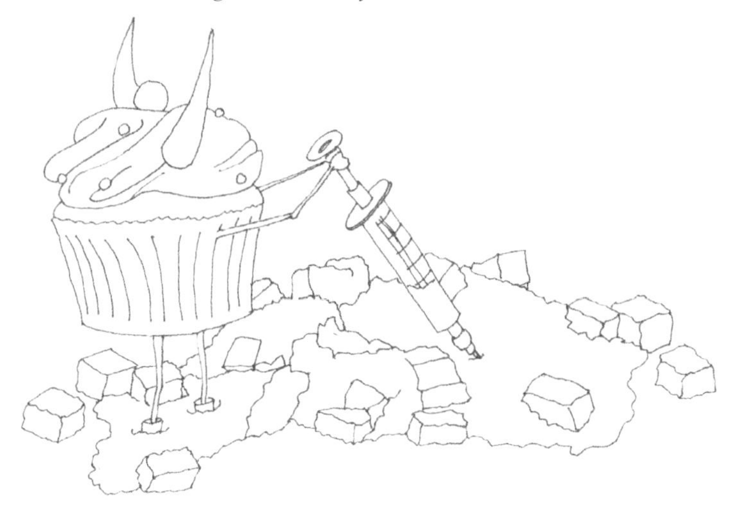

Chapter 5

Why sugar and refined carbohydrates have become such a problem

'Ancipiti plus ferit ense gula.' – 'Gluttony kills more than the sword. Wine has drowned more than the sea…'

Idiomatic translation of Ancient Latin proverb

There are at least six key drivers of the epidemic in sugar and refined carbohydrate consumption in the Western world. They are:

- Addiction
- Stress
- Love
- Propaganda
- Myths
- Intellectual idleness.

We shall look at each individually.

Addiction

I am a stubborn, greedy Westerner who loves food and good living. In order to change my diet and lifestyle I had to have extremely good reasons for doing so. Western diets are delicious, cheap and convenient, and their sugar and carbohydrate content makes them addictive. For me to make the necessary changes to my easy diet and lifestyle, not only did I have to have very good reasons to do so but also a clear understanding of the mechanisms by which the body manages fuel delivery mechanisms. Together, that gave me the intellectual imperative and the determination to put in place the most effective interventions. Having achieved this myself, I was in a much stronger position to help my patients who struggled with exactly the same issues that I too had struggled with.

In my experience, the single greatest bar to change is addiction. We are surrounded by temptations.

> *'I can resist everything except temptation.'*
>
> Lord Darlington in Act I, *Lady Windermere's Fan* (1892), Oscar Wilde (1854–1900)

Western lifestyles are inherently addictive and those addictions are freely and cheaply available. Every service station contains all the legal ones – sweets, chocolate, caffeine, nicotine, alcohol, gambling scratch cards and sex magazines. These are in addition to what some would describe as our addiction to fossil fuels.

The problem with addictions is that they give us pleasure – sometimes an 'upper', sometimes a 'downer'. We like uppers in the morning to fire us up for action – typically caffeine and sugar. We then control the downer which ensues, either with a further dose of upper, or we add in another addiction, such as chocolate, nicotine, alcohol, cannabis or other such. These are just the social addictions. We have many prescription addictions, such as SSRIs and other antidepressants, and major and minor tranquillisers. Indeed, I see life as an addictive ladder which starts with milk, sugar and refined carbohydrates, progresses on to caffeine and chocolate, and then to nicotine and alcohol, which take their toll during the younger teens. Some progress to cannabis, heroin, Ecstasy and other illegal, and so-called 'legal', highs. At some stage in life (if the imbiber has survived!) it is recognised that these addictions are doing no good at all and, in the 'strong minded', or perhaps more accurately in those with the help, resources and knowledge to make the changes, the process reverses. However, it is generally not recognised that sugar is perhaps the worst and most pernicious addiction and this is, chronologically speaking , the first and last addiction and the one which is hardest to kick. Indeed, I have reason to believe sugar addiction is as damaging as smoking tobacco.

One addiction leads to another, especially for those people who are natural addicts (I know – I am one such myself). It is often easiest to cut out addictions completely – rationing does not work. Most smokers cannot have just one cigarette a day – they have to give up completely, not just cut down. Staying clean from all addictions is much easier if all addictions are cut out – that includes sugar and refined carbohydrates (so-called junk food). Alcoholics know that complete abstinence is the only way to sobriety. Oscar Wilde summed up this facet of addiction when he said:

> *'A cigarette is the perfect type of a perfect pleasure. It is exquisite, and it leaves one unsatisfied.'*
>
> *The Picture of Dorian Gray* by Oscar Wilde (1854–1900)

And we all know what happened to Dorian Gray – stabbed in the heart by his own hand, his face and figure withered and decrepit!

However, if addictive substances can be used occasionally and judiciously to enhance a social occasion, then I have few concerns – I find that jokes are much funnier after a pint of (especially, dry) cider and, as *Reader's Digest* regularly detailed, laughter is the best medicine.

My daughter Ruth spotted the following in the *Telegraph*. She sent it to Sandi Toksvig, who read in out on Radio Four's *The News Quiz*:

> *'A man was kerb crawling in a red light area when his car was apprehended by a police officer. He was asked about the identity of the scantily clad female occupant of the passenger seat. "Oh," he said… "This is an old family friend that we have known for years … but for the life of me, I just cannot quite remember her name." The officer suggested that he use his mobile phone to telephone his wife to see if she could help him to recall the name. The offer was declined.'*

The problem is that great things have been achieved through addiction. These include the work of great artists, industrialists, musicians, writers, politicians, celebrities and comics, such as Howard Hughes (opiates), Oprah Winfrey (crack cocaine in her 20s), Charles Dickens, Ernest Hemingway, Pyotr Ilyich Tchaikovsky, Vincent Van Gogh and Edgar Allan Poe (alcohol), Marilyn Monroe (barbiturates), Samuel Taylor Coleridge (laudanum), Stephen King (Valium and Xanax – now recovered but does admit that he simply doesn't remember writing some of his novels), Jamie Lee Curtis (prescription painkillers, now recovered), Elizabeth Taylor (alcohol and painkillers), Robin Williams (cocaine and alcohol) and many others. Indeed, the 'idea' that addiction can lead to great things is so engrained in our culture that writers often have their main characters as addicts – Sherlock Holmes (cocaine) and even in the TV series, *House*, the lead, played by Hugh Laurie, is a Vicodin addict. William Pitt the Younger (British Prime Minister 1783-1801 and 1804-6) drank large amounts of port and probably died from liver failure. The British Empire was driven by addiction – trade for sugar, rum, coffee, tea, tobacco, wine, opium and others. The British Navy survived on a daily tot of rum and sailors put up with massive deprivations for their daily tot.

The rum ration, otherwise known as the 'tot', was one-eighth of a pint and was given out to each sailor at 12 noon. Petty Officers and more senior ranks were given neat rum, whereas for others it was diluted with two parts of water, making three-eighths of a pint of what was known as 'grog'. The rum ration was kept in, and served from, a specific barrel. Generally this barrel was highly decorated, made of oak, with brass bands and was emblazoned with brass letters spelling out, 'The Queen, God Bless Her'. The rum itself was sometimes referred to as 'Nelson's blood'. It is thought that this reference derives from the fact that following victory at the Battle of Trafalgar, Nelson's body was preserved in rum to facilitate its transportation back to England. It was in fact discovered, upon arrival in England, that some thirsty sailors had drilled a hole in the bottom of the cask and drunk all the rum! On 31 July 1970, the Royal Navy phased out the daily rum ration. This decision was much debated in the Houses of Parliament, especially by one Mr James Wellbeloved (MP for Erith and Crayford), an ex-Royal Navy man himself, and who, in the course of the debates, offered his fellow Parliamentarians 'sippers' and 'gulpers' of rum.[11]

In short, addiction is short-term gain and long-term pain for the imbiber (and often for the imbiber's friends and family), but cultural gain for humanity!

Finally, we are extremely skilful in rationalising our addictions, as the following internet meme illustrates:

'I've got salad for supper.
Actually a fruit salad.
Well, mostly grapes.
OK all grapes.
Fermented grapes.
Wine.
I've got wine for supper.'

Stress

We use addictions to cope with stress because they mask its symptoms. However, this is a potentially dangerous ploy because symptoms are present for very good reasons – they protect us from ourselves. Stress is the symptom we experience when the brain knows that we do not have the reserves to deal with demand. These demands may be financial, mental, physical or emotional, nutritional or infectious, allergic or inflammatory – all are energy-demanding and are made worse by lack of time. Stress is very unpleasant. In the short term we can gear up activity and energy delivery mechanisms to cope with it – the adrenal glands do this by producing adrenaline for short-term stress, cortisol for medium-term stress and DHEA for long-term stress. However, unremitting long-term stress results in chronic fatigue as the body protects itself from itself by stopping us from doing things, forcibly. This is essential – if total energy demand exceeds energy delivery, we die. This I suspect is what happened to the first marathon runner ...

> *'... Philippides, the one who acted as courier, ... brought the news of victory from Marathon and addressed the magistrates in session when they were anxious how the battle had ended; "Joy to you, we've won," he said, and there and then he died, breathing his last breath with the words "Joy to you".'*
>
> *A History of the Marathon Race 490 BC to 1975 (PDF)* John A Lucas, Pennsylvania State University & Los Angeles 1984 foundation. Retrieved 2012-04-08

Addiction masks unpleasant stress symptoms. Soldiers fighting in the Thirty Years War used alcohol for its believed warming properties on the body in cold weather and its calming effects before battle – these soldiers had noted the bravery-inducing effects of 'Jenever's Liquor' (gin) on Dutch soldiers and dubbed it 'Dutch Courage'.

'Alcohol is a good servant but a bad master.'

Old English proverb

Love

We feed our loved ones the things we love to eat and which give us an addictive hit. We now see children with metabolic syndrome – some are overweight, fatigued, mentally dull, anxious and 'ugly'. Some are hyperactive, irrational, obsessive compulsive, bad-tempered, turning into young offenders and tomorrow's criminals. Eating disorders, such as food faddiness, anorexia and bulimia, abound. Sexual maturity comes early and childhoods are lost. Recently reported was the youngest recorded case of type 2 'adult onset' diabetes – in a three-year-old, who weighed 35 kg (5 stone 7 lb, or 77 lb).

We feed our pets with carbohydrates – biscuit, rusk and tinned foods full of cereal. Our dogs and cats love these foods, and gobble them up, because they too get an addictive hit. This is resulting in epidemics of human diseases in pets – obesity, diabetes, fatigue, cancer and premature death. Garfield is an obvious example of a cat with metabolic syndrome and his jokes epitomise the problems of his condition – fatigue, carb addiction, foggy brain, inability to exercise, with no get up and go in the mornings, especially on Mondays! Garfield admits that his favourite sort of dog is a hotdog. Clearly he has never met Nancy, the carnivorous Patterdale terrier, and expert ratter, with whom I share a home.

Propaganda

For decades, we have been mis-sold poor dietary advice which says carbohydrates are good, and fats are bad. WRONG! This advice has been further driven by the food industry for several reasons:

- Sugar and fast carbs (junk food) are addictive – what better way to sell a product than get your punters addicted to it?
- Carbohydrate-based products are cheap to make but readily converted into expensive ones. A tonne of potatoes averages at about £100, but a tonne of potato crisps costs about £15,000.
- Sugar is a preservative. This means cheap carbohydrate snacks can sit on supermarket shelves for months; by contrast, fats, meats and vegetables go off quickly. Short 'sell by' dates are harder to manage and therefore cost more.
- By dint of doing simple calorie counts, sugars can be dressed up to appear as 'low calorie' and therefore we believe it is okay to eat more. But the calorie system is seriously flawed and ignores the metabolic controls that determine how calories are stored and burned. As a system of weight loss, calorie counting only works through starvation, with all the symptoms of such – namely, fatigue, foggy brain, depression and feeling cold. Only the very strong-minded can sustain a carbohydrate-based calorie-controlled diet – I know I can't!

Meanwhile, we are told that artificial sweeteners are a 'healthier' option, but as used in 'low calorie' products they are also addictive. They initially satisfy the brain's immediate desire for sugar. However, the brain is intelligent and has learned that a sweet taste will be followed by a sugar rush. I suspect that in anticipation of such the body initiates the hormonal mechanisms that usually follow: insulin is poured out, making blood sugar drop, in response to which adrenaline is poured out and the symptoms of hypoglycaemia are switched on. Artificial sweeteners keep the blood-sugar rollercoaster rolling and further drive metabolic syndrome. The high levels of insulin block keto-adaptation and fat burning. The body suffers severe fuel delivery problems, with neither sugar nor ketones being available to mitochondria for burning.

Biased information is everywhere. We like to believe that the facts and opinions offered by highly educated men and women (often described as 'scientists') dressed in dark suits or white coats are independent and based on good research. Nothing could be further from the truth. Indeed, it is my experience that the more 'education' received, the more likely is that person to toe the Establishment line. Worse still, these so-called 'independent minds' are as susceptible as any to the corrupting influence of money.

Myths

Myths have been burned into the national psyche:

- Myth one – 'High-fat diets cause high cholesterol which causes arterial damage and heart disease.' Even the doctors believe this nonsense despite there being not a shred of evidence to support it. They believe it because it makes for intellectually easy work. The pharmaceutical companies further encourage the fat myth since a simple money-making solution results – take statins! Even Dr Mosley, medical doctor and author of *The FAST Diet* has toed this line in the past, but has since said, 'I was wrong – we should be feasting on FAT.'
- Myth two – 'Eat your five a day of fruit and vegetables.' Growers also wish to sell addiction and achieve this by developing fruits and vegetables which are increasingly sweet. (Craig has to hunt high and low for his treasured occasional treat of bitter raspberries). Fruits spike blood sugars and are as addictive as sugar. The fruit-sugar fructose is even more pernicious than other sugars

because it inhibits the enzyme glycogen phosphorylase and so prevents the glycogen sponges (see page 225) from squeezing dry. Modern vegetables are low in the bitter but desirable plant nutrients such as carotenoids, ellagic acid, flavonoids, resveratrols, glucosinolates and so on. We need to start off by eating five portions of vegetables a day then move on to organic and ancient varieties grown in a soil where mineral levels have been corrected.

- Myth three – 'An apple a day keeps the doctor away.' Primitive man's idea of an apple would be a crab apple – good for flavouring a dish, but with minimal effect on blood sugar. Again, Craig used to scrump crab apples from the neighbour's garden opposite but these trees are no longer there – the humble crab apple is out of fashion. (Craig's note to Her Majesty's Law Enforcement Agencies – this offence is, in my opinion, now time limited.) Modern, intensively grown apples high in fructose and chemical residues and low in antioxidants are highly damaging. Concentrated fruit juice is even worse.
- Myth four – 'The food pyramid,' which features carbs at the base, rising to fats at the apex. This is an intellectually risible concept which has no base in science, is evolutionarily incorrect and biologically implausible. The School Food Standards guide for 2015 (produced with funding from the Department of Education, Defra and Public Health England, the Rothschild Foundation, the Sainsburys Charitable Trusts, and other trusts) lists, among other things, the following requirements for school meals: 'Three or more different starchy foods each week'; and it lumps its guidance for 'foods high in fat' and 'foods high in sugar' together, treating them as equal evils.[15] This re-enforces the food pyramid myth and embeds it into our children's eating habits.
- Myth five – 'Sugar gives you energy.' Oh dear! If blood

sugar runs low, then fuel delivery to mitochondria is impaired. A rising blood sugar level provides a brief window of time when blood sugar levels are perfect, but then as blood sugar rises too high, energy delivery is again impaired. The energy boost from sugar only results if blood sugar is very low and is short-lived before becoming a cause of fatigue. We call these 'uppers' and 'downers'. I suspect it is the high levels of blood sugar inhibiting mitochondria which explain the fatigue many diabetics complain of – this is akin to running your car with the choke constantly pulled out.

Intellectual idleness

'Study invites study; idleness produces idleness.'

Roman proverb

Addicts specialise in rationalising their addictions. Doctors are amongst the worst addicts – it is regularly said that an alcoholic is one who drinks more than his doctor. It is hopeless for a regular addict to try to advise a regular addict as to how to change. Doctors themselves do not understand metabolic syndrome so how can they possibly help their patients? I found that I had to 'live the life of an addict' in order to advise my patients as to their addictions. I now feel able to 'lead' by example. As one of my patients commented to me as she observed a diabetic receiving dietary advice from the hospital dietician: 'How can one sphere advise another sphere how not to be a sphere?'

Humour is a much-employed strategy that people use to rationalise their addiction – many a lawyer or politician gets his way by using humour, as laughs trump logic. I recall a particularly boozy evening when, as he glugged his gin and french, a friend of my father's stated:

'The trouble with not waking in the morning with a hangover is that you know that's the best you are going to feel all day.'

Summary

Advising and encouraging people to make the substantial and difficult lifestyle changes necessary to reverse metabolic syndrome and diabetes is intellectually and emotionally hard work for the doctor. It is much easier to dish out the drugs to suppress symptoms and blame the patient for his or her unhealthy lifestyle. This intellectual strait-jacket is further encouraged by Big Pharma since symptom-suppressing drugs 'for life' make money, as do the massive incomes from drugs for heart disease, cancer and, the next major growth area, dementia. An irony of this is that many of the drugs used to treat metabolic syndrome, diabetes and complications of such (such as statins, beta blockers and thiazide diuretics) accelerate the underlying disease process to make things worse. For example, statins inhibit endogenous production of co-enzyme Q10 and so could be expected to accelerate the ageing process with its attendant risks of heart failure, dementia and cancer.

Battling these six horsemen of the Apocalypse* is very tough, and most likely made much harder for you by your doctors who will, almost certainly, be supporting and encouraging these horsemen! Like King Agesilaus of Sparta, who, when asked why Sparta had no city walls, pointed at his warriors, and said, 'These are Sparta's walls', you must win this battle with your own determination alone.

*I am a woman in her 50s and so am allowed to take poetic licence to an extreme!

Chapter 6

How the body normally controls levels of sugar in the bloodstream

To be able to understand the prevention and treatment of metabolic syndrome and diabetes, we have to identify those mechanisms by which the body normally controls fuel delivery in the bloodstream and the effects when these mechanisms go wrong. Since the control of blood sugar is so vitally important to allow normal body functioning, there are several mechanisms in place. Too much sugar in the bloodstream is a problem; too little may also be a problem (if you are not keto-adapted); and swinging between the two is a problem. If we follow the passage of sugar through the body when the body is functioning normally, the chronological order for controlling its level in the blood is as described below, but, first, we should note that normal control of blood sugar involves:

- Sugars and carbohydrates in the diet, and how quickly these are digested and absorbed (fast carbs and slow-release carbs)
- The liver metabolic sponge (see page 225)
- The muscle metabolic sponge (see page 226)
- Insulin.

We then have the additional problems of controlling blood sugar which arise when there is an abnormal state of affairs, including:

- The fermenting gut and the alcohols this produces
- Thyroid malfunction
- Adrenal malfunction and chronic stress
- Metabolic inflexibility with poor keto-adaptation (that is, inability to switch from burning carbs to burning fat)
- Inflammation
- Insulin resistance.

The normal control of blood sugar

Sugar and carbohydrates in the diet

The complex sugars (sucrose, lactose) and carbohydrates that we consume are broken down in the gut and absorbed in the form of simple sugars (monosaccharides), such as glucose, fructose (fruit sugar) and galactose (from milk sugar, lactose). The ability of foods made up of these sugars and carbohydrates to raise blood sugar is described by what is called their 'glycaemic index' (GI). More formally, the glycaemic index of each food is a number associated with it that indicates its effect on a person's blood glucose (also called blood sugar) level. A value of 100 represents the standard – an equivalent amount of pure glucose. (For more detail see https://en.wikipedia.org/wiki/Glycemic_index). So, for example, fat has no carbohydrate content and has a glycaemic index of zero, but glucose is 100% simple carbohydrate and has a glycaemic index of 100. However, this index is determined by many factors and therefore is an imprecise measurement. These variables include:

- How refined the carbohydrate is (which determines the rate of absorption from the gut). Broadly speaking, 'junk foods', such as white bread and pasta, are refined carbohydrates with a high GI and are rapidly digested and absorbed.
- How fast the food is consumed. Gobbling of food or large

volumes of sweet drinks spikes blood sugar (and provides an addictive hit). Horace Fletcher (1849–1919, cause of death, bronchitis), also known as the 'Great Masticator', was famous for chewing each bite of food 100 times before swallowing: 'Nature will castigate those who don't masticate'. He attributed his good health, strength and endurance to this practice.

- Cooking of food. Cooking starts the breakdown of carbohydrate, so, for example, cooked potato has a high GI, while raw potato is indigestible. (The starches are contained within indigestible cellulose packaging.) The same is true of most pulses. So cooking food will begin the breakdown of carbohydrates, thereby increasing the GI.
- Combination with other foods. Fat and fibre both slow the rate of digestion and therefore absorption. So, combining high GI foods with fat and fibre will lower the overall GI.
- Alcohol. This is a solvent and carries sugars into the bloodstream rapidly, so beer has a higher glycaemic index than sugar, even though pure alcohol drops the blood sugar level. It does this by stimulating insulin secretion while inhibiting the secretion of glucagon (the hormone – chemical messenger – that takes glucose out of cells and into the bloodstream) – a real double whammy. So drinking alcohol with food will increase the overall GI.

The metabolic sponge in the liver

As sugars and all other products of digestion and fermentation (with the exception of fats) are absorbed from the gut, they do not pass directly into the systemic (whole body) circulation. Indeed, if they did, this toxic combination would cause such biochemical and immunological havoc that I suspect we would rapidly succumb. (Patients in liver failure, in whom precisely this happens, become acutely demented and fall unconscious.)

Except for fats, all the products of gut function are channelled into the vein known as the 'portal vein' which passes straight from the gut to the liver. The liver is responsible for sorting out this biochemically toxic soup. Furthermore, this demands a large amount of energy – at rest, the liver consumes 27% of all the energy produced in the body; this is as much as the heart and brain combined. I suspect some of my severely ill CFS/ME patients do not even have the energy for the liver to perform well – no wonder they suffer from foggy brains.

On the other hand, fats are absorbed into the lymphatics, a system of vessels which do not lead to the liver, but are poured directly into the bloodstream right next to the heart. I think this is a fine example of how safe fats are and how they do not damage blood vessels. They are non-toxic and, unlike all other products of digestion, do not have to pass to the liver to be detoxified.

A very particular problem for the liver is controlling levels of sugar (glucose, fructose, maltose, galactose, etc), which arrive from the portal vein. This sugar does not arrive from the gut in small, manageable amounts, but rather there is a tsunami of sugars that arrive after a high-carbohydrate meal. The liver cannot possibly use this wave of sugar immediately and so it employs what I call the 'glycogen metabolic sponge' – sugars are converted into glycogen and the glycogen is stored in the liver (and muscles – see below), a short-term pantry for sugar. The glycogen-pantry sponge quickly mops up sugar in the short term and so prevents sugar spilling over into the bloodstream where it would cause metabolic havoc. Indeed, I suspect this metabolic sponge is the most important way in which the body stabilises blood sugar levels; I say that because metabolically this is extremely efficient – much more so than using insulin. Employing insulin to bring blood sugar down is inefficient – the metabolic cost of producing insulin in the pancreas, which converts sugar into triglycerides and then deposits these into fat cells, is high. So is the metabolic cost of retrieving energy from fat. I suspect that insulin is a 'second line of defence' against sugar spikes from the gut and, from an evolutionary perspective, would only occasionally have been employed. I can see how it is therefore easy to 'exhaust' insulin and switch into diabetes. Modern Western man – and woman – is constantly invoking insulin to control blood sugar levels because s/he eats carbs at every meal and snacks between. No wonder the pancreas becomes exhausted.

However, for the glycogen sponge to be effective in mopping up sugar, it must be properly 'squeezed dry' and emptied between meals. We empty the liver's glycogen sponge by not snacking and having proper windows of time for fasting. As the body needs sugar, it is released in a very controlled way from the liver's glycogen sponge to precisely match demand. This requires the enzyme (chemical enabler) glycogen phosphorylase and is controlled by the hormone (chemical messenger) glucagon. Any problems with either of these result in impaired use of the glycogen sponge.

This flags up the very particular problem of fructose. For the biochemists, fructose inhibits glycogen phosphorylase – the enzyme that allows glycogen to be converted back into glucose. Essentially, what this means is that fructose stops our metabolic sponges from squeezing dry – we can no longer access this immediate energy source. This makes us particularly prone to falling blood sugars and all the dangerous hormonal responses to that – that is, the outpouring of adrenaline. Indeed, alcohol and fructose are especially dangerous for diabetics, particularly when they are already on medication to bring blood sugars down – a perfect storm to make blood sugar levels drop ensues. The triple whammy is:

1. Diabetic medication lowers blood sugar
2. Fructose prevents the metabolic sponge from releasing glycogen to correct the falling blood sugar level
3. Alcohol stimulates insulin release, which further drops blood sugar and inhibits fat burning.

Suddenly the body is unable to access any of its fuels; unconsciousness and death may result.

This problem is particularly severe in people with fructose intolerance. (Incidentally, they are also at increased risk of diabetes.)

The metabolic sponge in the muscle

A similar process occurs in muscle. We fill our muscle glycogen sponge after a meal and squeeze it dry through exercise.

When the glycogen sponges of the liver and muscle are full they hold about 380 grams of glycogen (more with training), which equates to approximately 1500 kCals of energy. Our basal (resting) metabolic rate consumes about 1270 kCals per day. Heavy exercise will consume 600-800 kCals per hour.

It is vital that between meal times we at least partially empty our liver and muscle glycogen sponges to be ready to mop up the flood of sugars from the gut that follow a carbohydrate meal. If these glycogen sponges are insufficient, systemic (whole body) blood sugar levels spike and that triggers our final line of defence against high blood sugars – namely, insulin.

So, for the muscle and liver metabolic sponges to work efficiently we need to:

- Restrict carbohydrates to one meal a day
- Not snack between meals
- Avoid excessive fructose (fruit, fruit sugar, corn syrup)
- Avoid alcohol and the upper fermenting gut (see Appendix 5, page 152)
- Have occasional windows of time for fasting, when the one carbohydrate meal of the day is missed or replaced by a fat and fibre meal. This squeezes completely dry the liver's metabolic sponge. We know this strategy reverses metabolic syndrome remarkably quickly.
- Supply the metabolic sponges with the necessary vitamins and minerals to function (see page 225).

Insulin

My guess is that if the evolutionarily correct diet were followed, together with evolutionarily correct exercise and irregular meals (primitive man would not have eaten a regular three-meals-a-day except during times of plenty), then insulin would rarely be brought into play. However, insulin would become necessary to cope with the autumn harvest as the fruit trees, roots, nuts and seeds ripened. These foods cannot be safely stored (without going rotten or being stolen). This is when a temporary period of metabolic syndrome would have had distinct evolutionary advantage in the past. Primitive man would have gorged himself on these carbohydrate windfalls, saturated his metabolic sponges, spiked his blood sugars and poured out insulin, which laid these sugars down as fats. These fats were an essential insurance policy, a pantry of fuel to allow winter survival – not just as a fuel but also as a warm, insulating layer of flesh. Metabolic syndrome allowed women to store fuel for pregnancy and breast feeding. Female sex hormones further encourage this metabolic drive and would have been poured out as food supply improved. Short windows of time of metabolic syndrome would have become a very useful survival and reproduction ploy.

Once we are fat, we become lethargic, depressed and cold because we can afford to turn down energy production because of the insulating effects of fat. These are highly desirable calorie-saving metabolic interventions which again allowed primitive Man to survive a long and cold winter – effectively, we go into a state of mild hibernation as we get fat. Indeed, in primitive communities this ability to lay down fat for survival is a highly rated attribute.

Western diets put us into a metabolic state of chronic autumn, with chronically high insulin. Diabetes results when insulin too is finally overwhelmed.

Justin Hayward sings of his depression and lethargy at losing his love and aptly names his song *Forever Autumn*, instinctively associating his depressive feelings with the time of year when these are, evolutionarily speaking, 'normal'.

Control of blood sugar when things start to go wrong

Certain factors compromise our ability to control levels of glucose in our blood, adversely affecting the mechanisms that have evolutionarily been beneficial for the human body.

Fermenting upper gut

Our 'upper gut' consists of the oesophagus, stomach and small intestine. These are where digestion takes place, with fermentation (of fibre, that cannot be broken down by digestion) being restricted to the lower gut (principally, colon) in healthy individuals. It is *not* healthy for fermentation to take place in the upper gut.

By 'fermenting upper gut' I refer to infection of the stomach by *Helicobacter pylori* and/or 'candida' (various yeasts, causing the 'auto-brewery syndrome'), and/or small intestinal bacterial over-growth (SIBO). I suspect all these problems are much more common than generally believed and that even the relatively small amounts of alcohol production which result, along with bacterial 'endotoxins', can have profound effects on blood sugar control (see Appendix 5, The fermenting gut, page 152).

The upper gut should be near sterile thanks to stomach acid. Acid kills all microbes. This is a major line of defence against ferment and infection. However, if stomach acid is reduced (for example, by acid-blocking drugs such as PPIs – proton pump inhibitors – which work on the cells that line the stomach, reducing the production of acid), or overwhelmed by a large meal or large drink (such as pints of fruit juice or beer), there is a risk that carbohydrates will be fermented by microbes already in the upper gut. The cardinal symptoms of this are heartburn, reflux, wind, bloating and burping. As I have said, the products of the fermenting gut include various alcohols and other 'endotoxins'. As detailed above, alcohol stimulates insulin secretion and so blood sugar levels drop. Worse still, alcohol inhibits fat burning (see metabolic inflexibility, page 239) and so, again, fuel delivery mechanisms are impaired. The hypoglycaemic effects of alcohol manifest for up to 16 hours and I suspect that this explains why it is so disrupting to sleep. It has similarly dysregulating effects on the brain – as Falstaff famously said of alcohol:

> *'It ascends me into the brain, dries me there all the foolish and dull and crudy vapours which environ it, makes it apprehensive, quick, forgetive, full of nimble, fiery, and delectable shapes, which delivered o'er to the voice, the tongue, which is the birth, becomes excellent wit.'*
>
> Act IV scene iii of *Henry IV, Part 2* William Shakespeare (1564–1616)

Also see Appendices 4 and 5, The fermenting mouth and gut, pages 149 and 152.

Thyroid disease – too much and too little thyroid hormone

Thyroid hormones are an essential part of blood sugar regulation; they facilitate the release of glucose from glycogen stores in the liver (gluconeogenesis) and also encourage fat burning.

Thyrotoxicosis – too much thyroid hormone – has effects in its own right, and secondary effects on other hormones. One result is high blood sugar. It is a metabolically dangerous situation, with uncontrolled fat burning and acute weight loss, and in diabetics (who, for whatever reason, also develop thyrotoxicosis) this can trigger ketoacidosis. This is a serious medical emergency.

Conversely, hypothyroidism – insufficient production of thyroid hormones – has the opposite effect. It results in low levels of blood sugar. This is a much more common problem than thyrotoxicosis and it is becoming ever increasingly common. Indeed, consultant endocrinologist Dr Kenneth Blanchard estimates that 20% of all Western women are hypothyroid or borderline hypothyroid – with profound effects on metabolism.[24]

Hypothyroidism results in metabolic inflexibility (that is, inability to burn fat rather than carbs) and this worsens metabolic syndrome. Indeed, I suspect this is the mechanism by which we see weight gain in hypothyroidism. (Also see part 5 of Chapter 7: Ensuring normal thyroid function, page 86.)

Adrenal malfunction – too much and too little adrenal hormones

The adrenal glands are centrally involved in blood sugar regulation. We know this because if they fail (Addison's disease), blood sugar levels run dangerously low and this can kill the sufferer. Adrenal hormones are essential for life.

The adrenal glands are part of the body's energy delivery mechanism and I liken them to the gear box of our cars. They allow us to gear up energy production in response to stress. By stress I mean any situation that demands energy; our core requirements include hunting for food, hunting for sex, hunting for warmth, fighting infection and healing wounds from war or animal killing. However, all stress elicits the same hormonal response from the adrenal glands.

The adrenal glands gear up energy delivery in several ways – for example, they allow mitochondria (the engines of our cars, so to speak, see page 236) to increase output by up to 200% of normal production. A further mechanism is to improve fuel delivery to cells so that the mitochondrial engines have sufficient fuel to increase energy production. The adrenal glands allow us to sprint when we should be walking. However, this state of acute stress is not sustainable in the long term, which explains why in the short term a hit of adrenaline is so delightful, but unremitting stress so painful.

The adrenal glands must be set just right – too much and energy is wasted; too little and we have insufficient energy to escape danger, hunt and survive. The adrenal glands are how Nature carefully gears energy expenditure to energy demand so there is no waste; indeed, she has built in inertia – a natural tendency to idleness – which again is for purposes of energy conservation.

The adrenal glands are geared for acute stress, with an outpouring of the short-term stress hormones adrenaline and cortisol, which, in Nature, usually lasts minutes or hours. Adrenaline pushes fuel (sugar or ketones) from the bloodstream into cells so it is available for mitochondria to burn. In the short term, this makes blood sugar levels drop. In the medium term, cortisol then mobilises sugar from stores in the body to increase blood sugar levels. During this time, blood sugar levels may run high (especially if we do not 'burn off' this sugar with exercise) and there is potential for this to do damage in all the ways detailed above. The spikes in levels of adrenaline and cortisol are followed by increases in other adrenal hormones, such as DHEA, which balance up the metabolic changes in adrenaline and cortisol. (Both cortisol and adrenaline are catabolic, meaning they break down tissue. DHEA, on the other hand, is anabolic, meaning it builds up tissue. In the cascade of hormone synthesis within the body, cortisol leads to the production of DHEA. In this way, the metabolic effects of cortisol and adrenaline are balanced by the production of DHEA.)

Problems arise with chronic stress because this results in chronic and persistent high adrenaline and cortisol levels, high blood sugar with high insulin levels, leading to metabolic syndrome and diabetes.

The bottom line is that short-term windows of stress are good for us, but long-term stress is bad.

A useful test for poor adrenal function is the adrenal stress profile (ASP – see Appendix 9: Tests, page 171).

Metabolic flexibility and keto-adaptation

Metabolic flexibility (or keto-adaptation) reflects the ability of the body to switch so its fuel comes from fats instead of carbohydrates. 'Inflexibility' relates to the loss of the ability to do so. Marathon runners sometimes experience this problem and they describe it as 'hitting a wall'. Despite being fit, they suddenly fatigue. The reason for this is that they have squeezed dry their liver and muscle glycogen sponges but are metabolically unable to switch to fat burning. They are unable to continue running because they have no fuel supply.

This problem often occurs in people with metabolic syndrome, who run their bodies entirely on carbohydrates. When blood sugar levels suddenly drop, they are unable to access fat to burn – despite having plenty of it. This is because insulin levels are high and insulin is the single greatest factor in blocking fat burning. I suspect this occurs because there is an inherent 'metabolic inertia'. This results because the body sees carbohydrates as a desirable short-term fuel for at least two reasons. The first is that the energy required to utilise carbs is much less; it is metabolically cheap to burn sugar. By contrast, mobilising and spending fat costs more. I liken this to a miser who keeps all his money in his fat deposit account. He relies on his current account for day-to-day energy spending and will not draw on his fat savings. Our miser has metabolic inflexibility. This is an evolutionarily safe ploy – saving fuel has huge survival value. Indeed, I consider our energy reserves to be like a bank – but our bank must never go overdrawn, because death ensues. Again think of Philippides, who ran the first marathon – he ran 150 miles in the two days prior to his final marathon, plus the additional 27 miles, before he ran out of fuel and collapsed dead.

I suspect that constant eating and snacking means we do not exercise our metabolic sponges and therefore our ability to store glucose as glycogen declines. The glycogen sponge shrinks, making the problems of blood sugar control even worse. We know the opposite is true – exercise increases the capacity of our metabolic sponges.

Modern Westerners live with an abundant food supply but our metabolism remains in the Dark Ages. We are fat misers. High-carbohydrate diets and metabolic syndrome result in hormonal imperatives to lay down, and cling to, fat. Fat is our evolutionary metabolic comfort blanket.

Metabolic inflexibility is one of the most difficult hurdles to overcome in the business of reversing metabolic syndrome, losing morbid fat and treating and preventing diabetes. Switching into fat burning has become an essential survival ploy for Modern Man. However, like the ultimate miser, Scrooge, from Dickens' *A Christmas Carol*, this is a challenge worth meeting:

> *'But if the courses be departed from, the ends will change.'*
>
> *A Christmas Carol*, Charles Dickens (1812–1870)

We switch to burning fat when we are stressed, and that involves hormones from the thyroid and adrenal glands. I know this when I go team chasing – the adrenaline flows, the bowels empty, I cannot eat, I do not feel hungry and I lose about half a stone in weight. This reaction also made our ancestors more effective hunters by further improving the power/weight ratio.

The key is to make this 'good' stress rather than 'bad' stress. Good stress arises from having a goal in life – a horizon, which drives us forward. This was brought home to me by my uncle,

Dr Charles Dansie, at his 80th birthday (he loved making speeches):

> *'No matter how old we are or where we are in life, we all need a horizon that we can look at and work towards.'*

Those horizons include competition, being creative, music and singing, the arts, sporting occasions, social events, worship, public spectacles, caring and loving others, courting (something my daughters seem awfully good at but with no grandchildren resulting) – indeed, all those things that make for a rich, inspiring and fulfilling life.

Inflammation

Inflammation results when the immune system is activated; where this occurs, the cardinal symptoms are heat (*calor*), pain (*dolor*), swelling (*tumor*), redness (*rubor*) and loss of function (*functio laesa*). Think of a boil!

> *Dolor, calor, rubor* and *tumor* were first described and documented by Aulus Cornelius Celsus (c25 BC to c50 AD), a Roman encyclopaedist. With regard to *functio laesa*, it is not clear who first described and documented the fifth sign, but the majority of attributions have gone to Thomas Sydenham (1624–1689), an English physician, and Rudolph Carl Virchow (1821–1902), a German doctor, biologist, politician and pathologist (*Medical News Today*[16]).

There is a very particular vicious cycle whereby high levels of blood sugar drive inflammation and high levels of inflammation drive up blood sugar levels. I think of this as a pro-inflammatory fire which, once stoked, gains a momentum of its own. It is a potentially disastrous positive feedback loop. The mechanisms of this positive feedback loop involve nasty words that are not memorable, and not important to remember, such as cytokines, reactive oxygen species, oxidative stress and leptin resistance.

We live in a pro-inflammatory Western world – so much so that the normal ranges for inflammatory markers in the blood have changed substantially during my lifetime as a doctor. When I qualified in 1981, the normal reference range for an ESR (erythrocyte sedimentation rate – an inflammatory marker in the blood) was <5 mm Hg/hour. It now varies from lab to lab, but for many it is <20 mm Hg/hour and for some it is up to 30 mmHg/hour. The 'normal' ranges also increase with age; they should not. This increase simply reflects the increasing prevalence of metabolic syndrome over recent time.

Work by Caroline Pond (Department of Zoology, University of Oxford) showed that fat is laid down where the immune system is busy.[17] This makes good sense – the immune system (our standing army) is greatly demanding of energy and needs instant access to deal with infectious challenges. However, if the immune system is busy in the gut because of allergy and/or fermenting gut, fat is deposited there to make us apple-shaped – and being so is a marked risk factor for metabolic syndrome and diabetes.

We are seeing epidemics of inflammatory conditions, such as allergy (estimated by Allergy UK to affect one in three of the UK population) and autoimmunity (estimated to affect one in 20 of the UK population). These conditions are driven by metabolic syndrome and also themselves drive metabolic syndrome, giving another potentially disastrous positive feedback loop.

I suspect the major pro-inflammatory problems facing Westerners, in order of priority are:

- Diets high in refined carbohydrate – 'junk food'
- Powerful antigens – especially wheat protein and cow's milk protein
- Alcohol
- Trans fats – margarines, heated polyunsaturated oils (see

Appendix 3, Good fats and bad fats, page 144).

- Low intakes of antioxidant foods – vegetables, berries, seeds, nuts
- Products of the fermenting gut, such as bacterial endotoxins
- Micronutrient deficiencies, such as vitamins D, C, E and B complex, minerals such as zinc, magnesium and selenium, and lack of essential fatty acids
- Chronic lack of sleep
- Chronic lack of love and companionship
- Chronic stress
- Vaccinations
- Pollutants – heavy metals (aluminium and mercury are used in vaccinations as 'immune adjuvants' to switch on inflammation)
- Pesticides – agricultural, food residues, spray drift
- Silicones – from breast augmentation and other implants, such as stents and hernia meshes
- Prescription drugs – statins in particular
- Chronic infection.

People often ask me about red and white meat as drivers of inflammation. I can think of no biologically plausible mechanism by which this should be so.

Insulin resistance

Often in cases of type 2 diabetes, not only is blood sugar high, but so is insulin. One would expect the opposite – that is to say, diabetes should result from insulin deficiency. This phenomenon is called 'insulin resistance' – the body produces plenty of insulin but the cells of the body do not respond to it. What is so odd to me is that doctors clearly recognise this issue but have yet to ask the obvious next question: 'What is the cause of this insulin resistance?' I suspect we are back to the Romans – 'Idleness produces idleness,' and here it is idleness of curiosity, which I regard as the worst kind.

One cause is all of the above – that is to say, all the causes and problems of metabolic syndrome impair the effects of insulin; this is an obvious vicious cycle. However, there are two further causes, namely micronutrient deficiency and toxic stress.

- **Micronutrient deficiency**: Insulin needs some micronutrients as co-factors in order to have its effects. It is ineffective without chromium, zinc, magnesium, selenium, manganese, copper and vanadium, and possibly others. I cannot think of a vitamin which is not directly or indirectly involved with blood sugar control, including insulin resistance. In particular, the following are vital: vitamins B3 (niacinamide), B12 (methylcobalamin), B1 (thiamine), B5 (pantothenic acid), B6 (pyridoxine), B8 (inositol), C (ascorbic acid) and D, and probably also essential fatty acids.
- **Toxic stress**: Insulin can be blocked by other chemicals. This issue was flagged up following a release of toxic chemicals – namely, dioxins – into the atmosphere as a consequence of an explosion at Sveso in Italy in 1976. A study in 1998 showed that excessive incidence of diabetes followed in local people who had been exposed. These polluting dioxins had been absorbed by these local people and had resulted in insulin resistance.
- A paper by Lee et al, published in the *Diabetes Care* in 2006, looked at the levels of persistent organic pollutants (POPs – pesticides and volatile organic compounds) in the general population.[18] It found that those with the highest levels of pollutants compared with those with the lowest levels of pollutants were 38 times more likely to be diabetic. There was a *Lancet* editorial (Porta 2006[19]) which commented: 'This finding would imply that virtually all

risk of diabetes conferred by obesity is attributable to persistent organic pollutants, and that obesity is only a vehicle for such chemicals. This possibility is shocking.' We know that some metals, such as nickel and mercury, may cause insulin resistance. (See Appendix 7, page 157, for a list of the toxic causes of insulin resistance.)

Chapter 7

Prevention, treatment and reversal of metabolic syndrome and diabetes

'Prevention is better than cure.'

Desiderius Erasmus (1466–1536)

'The time for action is now. It's never too late to do something.'

Antoine de Saint Exupery (1900–1944 (presumed))

Having identified the mechanism of metabolic syndrome and diabetes, this gives us a clear strategy for treatment. This is as follows:

1. Reduce the carbohydrate load from the gut by
   a) eating a low GI diet (see page 75)
   b) avoiding a sugar rush or hit (see page 77)
   c) including more fat in the diet (see page 80)
   d) getting calories from vegetable fibre (see page 82)
   e) preventing the upper gut from fermenting (see page 82).
2. Activate the liver's metabolic glycogen sponge (see page 83) by
   a) only eating carbohydrates at one meal a day, and no snacking
   b) once a week missing out the one carbohydrate-based meal of the day; this squeezes the liver's metabolic sponge completely dry.
3. Activate the muscle metabolic glycogen sponge (see page 84) by exercising.

4. Prevent insulin resistance by
   a) taking nutritional supplements (see page 84)
   b) reducing the body's load of pollutants through heating and showering regimes (see page 85)
   c) avoiding drugs which induce insulin resistance (see Appendix 8: Causes of insulin resistance, page 165)
   d) avoiding drugs which induce metabolic syndrome, notably female sex hormones (the Pill and HRT) but also major tranquillisers such as chlorpromazine (UK trade name, Thorazine), clozapine (UK trade name, Clorazil), olanzapine and risperidone.
5. Ensuring good thyroid function (see page 86).
6. Normalising adrenal function (which declines with age – see page 93).
7. Identifying and preventing inflammation (see page 94).
8. Adopting strategies that encourage fat burning – this means addressing metabolic inflexibility (see page 239) to allow the body to run on ketones (so-called keto-adaptation).

The above strategies are so effective at reversing diabetes that one has to be very careful not to induce such low blood sugar levels that there is hypoglycaemia, unconsciousness and death. However, this only occurs when prescription drugs are being used, such as insulin or oral hypoglycaemics (for example, metformin or sulphonylureas) *and* the body has such severe metabolic inflexibility that it cannot switch into fat burning. In reversing established diabetes, continuous blood sugar monitoring must be done so that hypoglycaemic episodes can be flagged up before symptoms occur. Once keto-adaptation has been established, the risks of hypoglycaemia can be substantially reduced, if not abolished.

1. Reduce the carbohydrate load from the gut by

(a) Eating a low GI diet

The body is remarkably adept at obtaining its fuels from a variety of foods. Carbohydrates are not essential foods – we can survive without them. However, they are great life enhancers – in the short term they are rocket fuels for the body and brain, but they must be eaten judiciously. The fuel which actually enters mitochondria (the power stations in our cells) is acetate (via what is called the carnitine shunt, as acetyl-CoA). One can get to acetate from fat via ketones, from fermenting vegetable fibre in the gut via short chain fatty acids, as well as from protein and carbohydrates via glucose. We are led to believe that the only fuel mitochondria can use is glucose, but this is not true and indeed is *very* misleading.

When I recommend to people that they change to a low-carb diet, their immediate reaction is, 'Oh, so you mean high protein?' No, I mean get your fuel from fat and vegetable fibre and keep your protein intake the same. Too much protein will overload your liver, which will convert some back to sugar (this is called gluconeogenesis) and leave a potentially toxic nitrogen load.

Table 12 provides a guide as to which foods have a low 'glycaemic index' (GI). The lower the GI the more you can eat and vice versa. Avoid very high GI foods completely; they are too good at switching on addiction.

Table 12: *Foods grouped by their Glycaemic Index*

Zero to very low GI		Meat, fish, poultry, eggs, meat fats, and vegetable, nut, seed and fish oils. Water, black tea, black coffee.
Low GI	55 or less	Pulses, seeds, nuts, nut butters, most vegetables, mushrooms, salad, dark chocolate (at least 80%), berries.
High GI	56 or more	All cereals, even whole grains (wheat, corn, rye, oats, barley, rice, quinoa, etc) Whole fruits – tropical fruits, apples, pears, plums
Very high GI	70 and above	Fruit sugars, fruit juices, corn syrup, sugar, white rice, white bread, cornflakes, packet breakfast cereals, maltose, beer, cooked potato.

Staple foods should be zero or low GI, but just because a food is low GI does not mean you can eat it *ad lib*. High GI foods should be eaten just once a day – these are the foods that easily saturate our liver and muscle glycogen sponges (page 225) with glucose. Once a week we should have a day completely free from high GI – this ensures the glycogen sponge is fully utilised by being fully squeezed dry.

Fruit

Primitive man's idea of fruit would have been a crab apple. Fruit growers know we are sugar addicts and have developed fruits which are increasingly sweet in order to satisfy the addict in us. Worse, these fruits are available all year round. Worse still, they make up the Government's recommended 'five a day'. Even worse, we have fruit juices touted as healthy drinks which are simply concentrated sugars with none of the goodness from peel, pips and pith. These drinks are even given 'innocent' names.

Dairy products

Dairy products evolved to nourish young mammals. If young mammals do not grow quickly they are eaten by sabre-toothed tigers. All dairy products contain growth promoters which can make us grow too quickly and too large. (It is known to increase IGF-1 [insulin-type growth factor 1] in the blood, which is highly anabolic.) Being tall, being fat and eating dairy products are all risk factors for cancer. Interestingly, the three known risk factors for juvenile-onset type 1 autoimmune diabetes are dairy products, vitamin D deficiency (lack of sunshine) and vaccinations. Since dairy products are one of the commonest allergens, and allergy is now estimated to affect 30% of the population, my view is that dairy products should not be staple foods but reserved for occasional treats. (The safest dairy product is butter as it is the milk protein [casein] and milk sugar [lactose] that are such a problem. Ghee is ideal since it is free of milk protein.)

(b) Avoiding a sugar rush or hit

Even with a well-emptied liver glycogen sponge, it is still possible to overwhelm the liver with a real sugar rush or hit. All the blood from the gut passes via the portal vein to the liver; however, if there is a large amount of sugar in a short window of time, some will spill over into the bloodstream. We know when this does not happen because we do not get a psychological hit from what we have ingested. Sugar addicts, and alcoholics, recognise this phenomenon and employ strategies to get around it. Some simply have to eat a large pudding over and above starters and main course. An obvious one is to eat/drink a large volume of high GI food or alcohol on an empty stomach. This is what the stressed stockbroker, journalist, author or publisher (present company excepted, of course) does at the end of a day – straight into a pub where two pints of beer are quickly downed to get the hit. So, one strategy for avoiding sugar rushes is to avoid such self-induced hits.

A 'Stock Exchange' themed bar has recently been opened in London. The concept is supposed to be 'all about having fun', but the technology behind it is quite serious. A pricing algorithm has been developed that is meant to mimic real-time markets. Effectively, if someone buys three beers then the price of that beer will rise and the price of other beers will fall. To illustrate the point above, the bar will be open from 5 pm to 2 am every Monday to Thursday and until 3 am on Fridays and Saturdays, thereby giving plenty of opportunity for the sugar rush hit at the end of a stressful day.

Another strategy to get a sugar hit is to avoid the gut completely. Sweets which are sucked and dissolve in the mouth allow sugar to pass directly into the bloodstream and bypass the liver's glycogen sponge. This has the added bonus of being inexpensive. (As a child I could eek out my thru'penny Sherbert Fountain by slowly sucking it over a whole afternoon for maximal benefit. Goodness only knows the damage this must have done to my teeth.)

In March 2014, the Royal Mint announced that a new design of one pound coin will be introduced in 2017, reprising the twelve-sided shape of the old thru'penny bit. The new one is designed to be more difficult to counterfeit.

Some alcoholics find that they can get a better hit by inhaling alcohol – the spirit is held in the mouth and inhaled air bubbled through so the spirit-evaporate passes directly into the lungs. Absorption is very rapid and the hit immediate (as any smoker can testify to). As a child I would watch attendees doing such at my parents' cocktail parties and could predict those whose words would shortly be slurred – including my parents! Indeed, double whammies can be achieved from very sweet alcoholic drinks. We call these cocktails.

So far we have discussed how to get a sugar hit, but this is undesirable because it will overwhelm the liver glycogen sponge. The advice is therefore to avoid getting these sugar rushes by:

- Avoiding sweet drinks completely – quench thirst with water only.
- Not snacking between meals.
- Not eating high GI foods on an empty stomach – especially not alcohol and sugar.
- Combining high GI foods with low GI foods. So, roast potatoes are better than boiled potatoes; the potatoes themselves are high GI but have been cooked in lard (or such like) which is low GI.
- Eating high GI foods slowly (remember the Great Masticator, page 56). Indeed, chewing stimulates the release of salivary endothelial growth factor which results in the gut being less permeable (leaky); this additionally protects against infections and allergies.
- Avoiding fructose (fruit sugar) – whilst listed as a lower GI food, fructose inhibits the enzyme that allows the glycogen sponges to work.
- Not using artificial sweeteners – the body is clever; if foods taste sweet it will anticipate a sugar rush and produce insulin in anticipation. This triggers the blood-sugar rollercoaster, blood sugar falls , adrenaline is poured out with hunger, sugar craving and anxiety resulting. This is a classical Pavlovian response.

HISTORICAL NOTE: During the 1890s, Russian physiologist Ivan Pavlov was looking at salivation in dogs in response to being fed, when he noticed that his dogs would begin to salivate whenever he entered the room, even when he was not bringing them food, because they were *anticipating* him bringing food. From this came the theories of classical conditioning – a learning process by which a neutral stimulus (in this case, entering the room, or, in his formal experiment, ringing a bell), when repeatedly paired with a second stimulus (being fed) comes to produce the response the second stimulus has, without the second stimulus being present.

(c) Including more fat in the diet

Fat is good for us. It is an excellent calorie-dense fuel. In the past this afforded huge evolutionary advantages. It allowed us to store energy to survive the winter and migrate to live away from the equator. It allowed us to become excellent hunters by making us clever and supplying us with an energy source.

The brain is largely made up of fat – indeed, a diet high in animal fats and seafood provided the raw materials to allow the brain to develop and grow bigger. Larger brains have the potential to make us clever and this clearly has huge survival value.

The evolution of human intelligence is a fascinating area. Some of the theories as to why intelligence is selected extend beyond the capability of being good hunters and providers, crucial as that aspect is. For example, good nutritional status confers better cognitive function and this may have been seen as a 'marker' of a good sexual mate by the inference of having access to a good food supply. Also, there are medical and social theories that intelligence was correlated with disease resistance (to illnesses that caused mental decline) and therefore intelligence was seen as desirable for that reason. Last, but not least, the creative ability that often comes with intelligence confers sexual attraction and so this further enhances the selective nature of intelligence.

However, we humans were so successful as hunters not just because we were clever but also because we had better stamina than our prey animals. We could fuel our bodies with fat (which is light), and, furthermore, gaining fuel from fat, which is easily digested, meant we evolved small light-weight digestive systems. Compare this to a gorilla which has an enormous gut – he could not possibly hunt.

This light-weight, well-fuelled body meant we could run down deer, bison and antelope over several days and they would get exhausted before we did. They became exhausted first because they had to carry a huge gut around with them as they gained their fuel from vegetable fibre. This is heavy stuff, needing a huge fermenting vat of a stomach to extract fuel in the form of short-chain fatty acids. Indeed, this stamina-based hunting strategy is still used by other fat-loving predators, such as wolves chasing caribou.

In addition, fat gives us a much larger fuel tank for stamina. The glycogen sponge fuel tank can supply about 1700 kCal. By contrast, someone of normal body weight carries enough fat to deliver 140,000 kCals. This is evidenced by the work of Drs Stephen Phinney and Jeff Volek, [20] who train elite athletes to run on ketogenic diets with gold medal results.

In Nature there is no such thing as a bad fat. 'Bad fats' only arise when we heat poly-unsaturated fats or mono-unsaturated fats, or we hydrogenate them in the manufacture of margarine (see Appendix 3, page 144, for a full explanation).

Fat is important because as a food it cannot be fermented. How do I know this? I can leave a lump of lard in my fridge for months and it does not go off. The same is true for a bottle of oil. Eating fat helps prevent upper fermenting gut. So, more rules of the game are:

- Do not eat hydrogenated fats, as in margarine and 'spreads';
- Cook with saturated fats such as lard (any animal fat), butter or coconut oil;
- Use cold-pressed oils from plant sources at room temperature – do not cook with them.

See Appendix 3 (page 144) for a more biochemical explanation of these rules.

(d) Getting calories from fibre

Eat high-fibre foods, such as vegetables, nuts, seeds and pulses. Vegetable fibre is fermented in the large bowel by friendly bacteria to short-chain fatty acids (SCFAs). Up to 500 kCal of fuel a day can come from this source. As importantly, these SCFAs nourish the lining of the large bowel directly, and are also highly protective against bowel cancer.

(e) Preventing the upper gut from fermenting

Do all of the above – that is, eat a low GI diet, with carbs at just one meal a day, and fuel the body with fat and vegetable fibre.

In addition, take vitamin C to bowel tolerance (see below) last thing at night; the idea here is that vitamin C kills all bacteria, yeasts and, indeed, viruses. It is poorly absorbed which, for this purpose, is ideal. The idea is to take enough vitamin C to kill the millions of (potentially bad) microbes in the upper gut, but not enough to kill the billions and trillions of (good) microbes in the lower gut. Start with 2 grams at night, increase until there is slight diarrhoea, then reduce a little – that is what I mean by 'to bowel tolerance'. My bowel tolerance is 4 grams. Unlike all other mammals, and along with fruit bats and guinea pigs, humans cannot make their own vitamin C and most modern humans are deficient. Linus Pauling, winner of two Nobel prizes, became a champion of vitamin C for its anti-cancer, anti-ageing and protective effects against heart disease. (See Appendix 5 – The fermenting gut, page 152.)

I am no cook, but a few recipes are essential until supermarkets start to respond to the demands of this diet. I have chosen recipes which are delicious and provide an excellent substitute for yoghurt, double cream, bread and a crumble topping for puddings (see Appendix 1, page 134). You also need a great French dressing to enhance all salad and pulse dishes, together with a recipe to render fat and make the most delicious scratchings – a crunchy topping for any meat dish.

2. Activate the liver's metabolic glycogen sponge

This should be done by following the steps described next.

(a) Eat carbohydrates at only one meal a day – and no snacking

- No snacking – Snacking never allows your body's metabolic sponge to squeeze dry, so to speak. I suspect that the sponge can be 'exercised' to make it more effective. We know that physical exercise allows more storage of muscle glycogen and so it is biologically plausible that the same applies to the liver.
- Do not eat carbohydrates with every meal – Aim to eat high GI foods at just one meal a day. The idea here is that the liver's glycogen metabolic sponge can supply sugar for basal metabolism for about 24 hours, ergo it takes 24 hours to squeeze dry. The more the metabolic sponge is exercised, the more effective it will be at mopping up sugar from the gut.

(b) Go without starchy carbs for one day a week

Once a week, miss out the carbohydrate meal (or replace it with a fat and fibre meal); this squeezes the liver's metabolic sponge completely dry. Perhaps even once a week, have a day when you eat very little – say 500 calories in the day. This is the quickest way to reverse metabolic syndrome. Interestingly, it is a powerful stimulus to create more connections in the brain; this makes good evolutionary sense – when primitive man got hungry, he got clever and so became a better hunter. Dr Dale E Bredesen, a neurologist from California, reversed Alzheimer's in nine out of 10 patients with the above regime. He insisted his patients eat their meals within a 10-hour window of time so there was a 14-hour fasting period in every 24. His only failure was the one patient who could not stick to this regime.[21]

3. Activate the muscle metabolic glycogen sponge by exercising

The importance of exercise in blood sugar control is not that it burns up excess calories (one has to do a huge amount of exercise to achieve this), but because it exercises the glycogen sponge provided by the muscles and so increases the ability of this 'sponge' to stabilise blood sugar levels.

4. Prevent insulin resistance and improve insulin sensitivity

There are three key steps to improving insulin sensitivity.

(a) Take nutritional supplements

Modern diets are so deficient in micronutrients that everyone should be taking a Basic Package of nutritional supplements. There is much more about this in my book *Sustainable Medicine*, but the essentials are a good multivitamin, multi-minerals, essential fatty acids, vitamins C (to bowel tolerance) and D (5000 iu – international units – daily). We then have the 'bolt-on extras' of supplements which are essential for blood sugar control. These include:

- Zinc – 30 milligrams at night
- Chromium (also called 'glucose tolerance factor') – I often

prescribe 2 milligrams daily for two months to correct a deficiency, followed by a maintenance dose of up to 600 microgams daily, long term.

- Iodine – 1 milligram daily.
- Niacinamide – 500-1500 milligrams slow release daily.

(b) Reduce the body's load of pollutants

Reduce the pollutant load firstly by reducing exposure and secondly by increasing excretion. Appendix 8 contains a list of the commonest offenders. Pollutants may come from the inside world (from the fermenting gut – see above and Appendix 5) and also from the outside world (pesticides, volatile organic compounds and toxic metals). We live in an increasingly toxic world and to avoid them completely is impossible. The best we can do is to stay in equilibrium with them – at as low a level as possible. In this respect, heating and washing regimes are helpful. The idea here is that many of these toxins are fat soluble and volatile – that is, they bio-accumulate in fat, including fat under the skin. Getting hot evaporates ('boils') them off onto the lipid layer on the surface of the skin – from where they can be washed off. This may be another possible mechanism by which exercise protects against the development of metabolic syndrome and diabetes. Sauna-ing, far infrared saunas and Epsom salt baths in theory should work as well. See Appendix 9 (page 171) for tests to measure our body's load of toxins.

(c) Avoid particular prescription drugs

Certain prescription drugs induce insulin resistance, notably female sex hormones (the Pill and HRT), but also many others. See Appendix 8 (page 166) for drugs causing insulin resistance.

5. Ensuring normal thyroid function

Both an overactive thyroid (hyperthyroidism) and an underactive thyroid (hypothyroidism) can result in metabolic syndrome with abnormal and wobbly blood sugar levels.

We are currently seeing 'epidemics of thyroid disease, especially hypothyroidism' – these are not my words but rather those of Dr Kenneth Blanchard, consultant endocrinologist. He estimates that 20% of women in the Western world are hypothyroid. Hypothyroidism is a major risk factor for metabolic syndrome because the thyroid gland is responsible for our basal metabolic rate – that is, the amount of energy that we burn at rest. Being hypothyroid, therefore, puts us in chronic 'go slow' mode with a tendency to weight gain, chronic fatigue, foggy brain and depression.

Hypothyroidism has become very common for several possible reasons but I suspect the main ones are:

- chronic iodine deficiency
- greatly increased incidence of auto-immunity (roughly one in 20 of the population suffer from at least one autoimmune disease, of which the most common is hypothyroidism)
- viral thyroiditis (as a result of there being more viral infections than ever), together with
- toxic stress to the thyroid gland from fluoride, heavy metals, radioactive iodine 131 (from Windscale [now re-named Sellafield], Chernobyl and Fukushima) and other such pollutants; indeed, a list of those toxins that affect the thyroid gland is very similar to that which causes insulin resistance (see Appendix 8, page 165).

Unfortunately, the only people who receive thyroxin via the NHS are people who have primary thyroid failure with a TSH (thyroid stimulating hormone) level above 5 mIU/l. (TSH levels are measured in milli International Units per litre.) The actual levels of thyroid hormone (free T3 and free T4) are not routinely measured. This means many cases of secondary hypothyroidism due to poor pituitary function and tertiary hypothyroidism due to poor conversion of inactive T4 to active T3 are missed. This problem is compounded when clinical factors are ignored.

Essentially there are four reasons why UK citizens are not subject to 'best practice' with respect to prescribing thyroid hormones. All relate to the prescribing of thyroid hormone for underactive thyroid glands (hypothyroidism).

Reason 1: The threshold for TSH is set too high

When levels of thyroid hormones in the blood start to fall, the pituitary gland increases its output of thyroid stimulating hormone (TSH), which kicks the thyroid into life and increases output of thyroid hormones. If the thyroid gland starts to fail, this is reflected by levels of TSH rising. The question is, at what point should the prescription of thyroid hormones begin? The normal range for TSH in the UK varies enormously from one laboratory to another. This means in some locations in the UK a thyroid prescription would not be given until the TSH rises above 5.0 mlU/l.

As a result of research, the normal range for TSH in America has been reduced so that anybody with a TSH above 3.0 mlU/l is now prescribed thyroid hormones. This research has shown that people with a TSH above 3.0 mlU/l are at increased risk of arterial disease (a major cause of death in Western societies), insulin resistance (and therefore diabetes), inflammation and hypercoagulability (sticky blood). Indeed, there is a recommendation afoot in America to further reduce the threshold for prescribing to 2.5 mlU/l.

What is completely illogical is that in the UK the target TSH level for patients who are actually on thyroid replacement therapy is often stated as being less than 2 mlU/l, or even less than 1.5 mlU/l. This is a ridiculous anachronism given that prescription is not recommended until levels exceed, say, 5.0 mlU/l. So, someone could have a level of 4.0 mlU/l and not be receiving thyroid replacement therapy (because their level is not above 5.0 mlU/l), whereas if someone was on thyroid replacement therapy, a level of 4.0 mlU/l would be considered much too high and would need to be brought down to below 2.0 mlU/l, or even 1.5mlU/l.

We should amend the threshold for prescribing thyroid hormones to 3.0 mlU/l, or better still, 2.5 mlU/l.

There is a further inconsistency in BTA (British Thyroid Association) guidelines. The level of thyroid hormones in pregnancy is critical for foetal development. For pregnancy the target for TSH is a level below 2.5 mlU/l. Furthermore, requirements during pregnancy increase, so thyroid function should be checked every three months. What is the logic of only prescribing thyroid hormones to a non-pregnant woman with a TSH of above 5.0 mlU/l but if pregnant the prescribing of thyroid hormones would start when levels exceed 2.5 mlU/l?

Dr Kenneth Blanchard states that reliance on a TSH reading to diagnose hypothyroidism is the biggest single medical error of modern times. It has resulted in millions of people missing out on this safe, life-transforming and disease-preventing treatment.

Reason 2: Confusing population normal range with individual normal range – they are not the same

The population normal range for levels of thyroid hormones in the blood is not the same as the individual normal range. We differ as individuals in our biochemistry as we differ in our looks, intelligence and morphology (structure). This biochemical variation should be taken into account when it comes to prescribing thyroid hormones.

The population normal range of free T4 (thyroxine in the

blood) is 12–24 pmol/l (picamoles per litre). A patient, therefore, with blood levels of 12.1 would be told he or she was normal because the level is within the population reference range, but actually that person's 'personal normal range' may be higher than the background 'population normal range'. He, or she, may feel much better running a high T4 level of, say, 24 pmol/l – that is, nearly twice as much, but still within the population reference range. Consultant endocrinologist Dr Antony Toft, in the first edition of his book for the BMA (British Medical Association), *Understanding Thyroid Disorders*, states that some people do not feel well until their T4 is running at 30 pmol/l.[22]

Research done originally in the UK, and now repeated in America, clearly shows that the individual normal range of thyroid hormones is not the same as the population reference range.[23] As the authors Koulouri et al say, 'In any given individual T4 and T3 concentrations remain relatively constant throughout life, and reflect the "set-point" of the hypothalamic-pituitary-thyroid (HPT) axis in that individual.' In order to find out who is outside the population range, patients have to be assessed clinically (that is, for clinical signs and symptoms of thyroid disease) as well as biochemically. This means assessing levels of fatigue, for example, and signs such as thinning hair and eyebrows. In actual UK clinical practice this is rarely done except by a few physicians conversant with this issue, yet it is the subjective clinical judgement that needs to be made in order to diagnose these individuals.

'Everything that can be counted does not necessarily count; everything that counts cannot necessarily be counted.'

Internet Meme wrongly attributed to Albert Einstein

Reason 3: Some people have poor conversion of the relatively inactive thyroxin (T4) to the biologically active T3

In theory, if patients have been shown to be hypothyroid, then all their symptoms should be improved with synthetic sodium thyroxin. In practice, this is not always the case; there is no doubt that clinically some patients feel very much better taking biologically identical hormones, such as natural thyroid (a dried extract of pig thyroid gland which is a mix of T4 and T3). Indeed, before synthetic thyroid hormones became available, all patients were routinely treated with natural thyroid. (The purity and stability of these preparations have been long established, indeed much longer established than synthetic thyroxin.)

Part of the reason why people feel better taking natural bio-identical hormones is that some people are not good at converting T4 (which is relatively inactive) to T3 (which is biologically active). However, this does not explain the improvement in every case. It is difficult to explain why there should be an additional effect, but for many people it is the difference between drinking cheap plonk and good quality claret. The alcohol content is the same, but the experience completely different!

Reason 4: Some people have thyroid hormone receptor resistance

We can infer this problem (receptor resistance) because some people only feel well when taking very high doses of thyroid hormone. Blood tests may be off the scale, but clinically there are no signs of thyrotoxicosis (thyroid excess). We can only explain this phenomenon in terms of thyroid hormone receptor resistance – that is to say, something is blocking the receptor. There is a detailed discussion of this in Paul Robinson's book *Recovering with T3: my journey from hypothyroidism to good health using the T3 thyroid hormone.*[25]

Conclusion

The proper diagnosis of hypothyroidism requires blood tests, the clinical picture *and* the patient's response to treatment. Often, the only way to secure a diagnosis of hypothyroidism for some is a trial of thyroid hormones. It is a sad fact that there are very few doctors who diagnose hypothyroidism in this way and, therefore, there are thousands, if not millions, of people who are suffering as a result of borderline hypothyroidism which passes unrecognised and untreated, causing untold misery.

The essential minimum range of blood tests to start the diagnostic process includes a free T3, free T4 and TSH reading. Ideally, one would also measure thyroid antibodies. These tests can now be done on a finger-drop sample of blood but the request must be made by a doctor and the results received by a doctor. Unfortunately, our NHS will rarely measure levels of free T4 and free T3 and so these tests must be done privately (see Appendix 9, How to access tests to further investigate metabolic syndrome and diabetes, page 171).

Treatment of hypothyroidism

If the clinical picture is suggestive (the commonest presentation is with metabolic syndrome that does not respond to diet and all other recommendations in this book) and the blood tests show that there is biochemical scope, then a trial of thyroid hormones is called for. Any such trial needs careful clinical monitoring, with checks of pulse and blood pressure together with monitoring of signs of over-treatment (see 4 below). The rules of the game are:

1. Start with very modest doses, such as 25 micrograms (mcg) of thyroxin (T4) once daily. Increase the dose every two weeks by 25 mcg increments to 75 mcg daily. At this point, wait four weeks, then re-check the above blood tests. This gives us two points on the graph (if we were

plotting dosage against serum thyroid hormone T4 levels) and that, together with the clinical picture, gives an idea of how much more, if any, thyroxin is required. For many, it is the last 25 mcg that makes the world of difference. Some people do not feel well until their free T4 is running above the upper limit of the reference range. (Please note that, just as TSH reference ranges have risen, reference ranges for T4 have fallen with time in parallel with our current epidemic of hypothyroidism – some NHS reference ranges for T4 are as low as 7-14 pmol/l.)

2. Monitor blood pressure and pulse. These should normalise at about 120/80 mm Hg, with a pulse of 60-80 beats per minute, depending on the person's level of physical fitness.
3. Continue to increase the dose until the individual feels well, so long as blood pressure and pulse rate remain normal and there are no symptoms of overdosing. Most people need between 75 and 200 mcg to be well, and physically big people need more (up to 300 mcg), whereas smaller people need less (perhaps as little as 25 mcg).
4. If there are any signs of overdosing, then reduce the dose at once and re-check the blood levels. The symptoms of overdosing include being anxious, irritable and unable to sleep, and tremor – similar to having drunk many cups of strong coffee!
5. Repeat the blood tests to make sure that the person is staying within or close to population reference ranges.
6. If there is no clinical benefit, consider swapping to natural (Armour) thyroid. This has a lower proportion of T4 to T3. In humans, the ratio of T4 to T3 released into the blood is roughly 20 to one, whereas one grain of Armour Thyroid (about 60 mg of desiccated pig thyroid extract) contains about 38 mcg of T4 and 9 mcg of T3, a ratio of around four to one. Thus Armour Thyroid is more biologically

active because it contains more of the active T3 relative to the inactive T4 than is generally released into the blood. Roughly speaking, 75 mcg of thyroxin is equivalent to one grain of Armour Thyroid.

Because the effects of thyroid hormones are so profound – indeed, life changing – and there are so few doctors willing to step outside NHS and NICE guidelines and prescribe thyroid hormones in the above way, many people have worked this out for themselves and have taken matters into their own hands. They get their thyroid hormones and their tests online. Whilst this is less desirable than having one's treatment overseen by a doctor, it is more desirable than no treatment. This is a most unfortunate result of the dismal quality of current medical practice – much more of this in my second book, *Sustainable Medicine*.

Hypothyroidism is a miserable, life-threatening condition, which can be safely and effectively treated given the above rules. Thyroid UK is a charity which has been set up by people who have found themselves in this situation, to help others (see page 131).

6. Normalising adrenal function (which declines with age)

If we think of our body as a car (a metaphor I find useful in looking at energy delivery in my other books), the adrenal glands are the gear box and allow us to match energy demand with energy delivery. As we age, the function of the adrenal glands declines and I suspect that declining levels of adrenal hormones accounts for what I call 'acquired metabolic dyslexia'. It may be that judicious use of adrenal hormones will improve energy delivery mechanisms and slow the ageing process.

The standard clinical test for adrenal dysfunction is what is called a 'short synacthen test' which measures cortisol levels in the blood following an injection of ACTH, a hormone that gives the adrenal glands a huge kick. However, this is a blunt tool. Whilst it may be very helpful in diagnosing Addison's disease (a condition where the adrenal glands have been destroyed, usually by autoimmunity) it does not pick up mild adrenal fatigue.

A more helpful test is an 'adrenal stress profile'; this measures levels of two adrenal hormones – namely, cortisol and DHEA – in a salivary sample. I like this test because it can be done at home and, therefore, results are not skewed by acute stress. Also, it measures the free hormone available in the blood and so results are not fudged by the problem of protein binding (this is an issue with blood tests).

What I very commonly see is adrenal fatigue with poor output of cortisol and/or DHEA. To treat this I recommend pregnenolone 25–50 milligrams sublingually daily. Pregnenolone is the most upstream of all adrenal hormones – that is, all others are derivatives of it. I am still collecting results, but my clinical experience so far is that pregnenolone is helpful and restores normality (clinically and biochemically). I suspect a small dose of pregnenolone as we age is helpful generally to slow the ageing process – indeed, pregnenolone has also been dubbed the 'memory hormone'.

7. Identifying and preventing inflammation

Inflammation occurs when the immune system is busy and this may be due to infection, allergy, autoimmunity, or healing and repair. Diabetes often shows up with an acute chest or urine infection as blood sugar levels run higher than usual and this encourages infection – microbes love to ferment sugar. Many doctors who deal with patients who are allergic recognise that allergy can result in high or low levels of blood sugar. There is a particularly vicious cycle with sugar and inflammation because each drives the other. Indeed, the ketogenic diet – see later (page 109) is markedly anti-inflammatory.

It is beyond the scope of this book to list all the causes of inflammation, but putting in place my recommended Basic Package of: Stone Age, low GI diet; taking nutritional supplements; ensuring good quality sleep; exercise; sunshine; and love and laughter will address many causes. Much more information is available in my book *Sustainable Medicine*.

8. Strategies to encourage fat burning

Fat burning can occur when all the above has been put in place. However, the greatest single inhibitor of fat burning is insulin.

The body will only access fat when it has squeezed dry its liver and muscle glycogen sponges. I think of fuel as money with fat representing our deposit account and carbohydrates our current account. We like to use our current account for everyday expenditure and dip into the deposit when the system is stressed. In Nature the two biggest stressors would have been hunting and sex. Indeed, my ex, Nick Myhill, used to cull deer for the Forestry Commission. He routinely weighed fallow bucks, entire and gralloched (gutted), before, during and after the rut. During rutting, the proportion of gralloch fell markedly as the bucks stopped eating and spent all their energy on fighting and sex. They ran their metabolism on fat. After the rut, they would start eating again but their total body weight would have fallen so dramatically that winter survival was seriously compromised.

'Hunting' for modern Western societies now encompasses a huge range of activities from the physical, such as sports, to the cerebral pleasures of music and performance. All such are enhanced by competition.

It is absolutely vital for the established diabetic to learn fat burning. This is because doing such is highly protective against hypoglycaemia. Indeed, one paper, by Drenick et al as long ago as 1972, showed that people who were keto-adapted could run their blood sugar as low as 0.5 millimoles per litre (mmol/l) without experiencing any serious symptoms of hypoglycaemia.[26]

A very useful tool is a glucose/ketone meter (such as Freestyle Optium – see page 132) which tells you when you are burning fat. Start off with just measuring glucose because you will not switch into fat burning mode until your blood sugar falls below 5 mmol/l (by doing all the above). As keto-adaption occurs, blood ketones will rise. A very low carb diet (<50 grams per day) will result in blood ketones of 0.5-3.0 mmol/l. Fasting will result in levels of 5-8 mmol/l. Once the diabetic can run on fat, he/she can safely run blood sugar levels much lower *and* be protected from hypoglycaemia.

Serious diabetic ketoacidosis (see page 234) gives ketone levels of 10-25 mmol/l – this is a medical emergency requiring hospital admission. This only occurs in type 1 diabetes when insulin is very low or absent, and glucose and fat burning, normally restrained by insulin, consequently becomes very high, and must be differentiated from ketosis (see page 234), which is safe and desirable.

How to incorporate all the above into your daily life

Table 13 shows a typical daily schedule that incorporates all the above recommendations.

Table 13: *Daily plan for avoiding metabolic syndrome and diabetes*

Time	Action	Mechanism
Rising	Drink a large glass of water.	To rehydrate. Do not use tea or coffee, which dehydrate.
	Exercise – sufficient to get hot – this may mean over-dressing.	You should exercise enough to get short of breath and to sweat. (1) Warming the subcutaneous fat 'boils off' pollutants onto the lipid layer on the surface of the skin. (2) Exercise squeezes dry the muscle metabolic sponge (see page 226).
	Hot shower – but take care with chemical cleaners and cosmetics, and with deodorants, many of which contain aluminium.	(1) Wash off toxic chemicals from the skin. (2) Use transdermal minerals on the skin to reduce bacteria on the skin and nourish the body.
Breakfast	Fry up – bacon, sausage, black pudding, chops, belly pork, steak, eggs, mushrooms, tomato, linseed 'bread' slices fried in lard, beans. Cook with lard.	(1) Power the body with fat and fibre. (2) Don't start the blood-sugar rollercoaster. (3) Squeeze dry the liver glycogen sponge. (4) Don't feed the fermenting gut or the fermenting mouth with carbs.
	Supplements: Multivitamin; omega-6 and omega-3 oils; chromium 600 micrograms; iodine 1 millgram; vitamin D3 5000 iu.	Improve insulin sensitivity.

Time	Action	Mechanism
	Supplements: Multi-minerals and glutathione 250 milligrams.	This combination is good for excreting toxic minerals such as lead and mercury.
Morning	No snacking. Quench your thirst with water. Black coffee or tea.	Squeeze dry the liver glycogen sponge.
Lunch	Low GI foods. Cold meat, salad, vegetables, pulses, coconut-milk yoghurt, berries, dark chocolate.	(1) Power the body with fat and fibre. (2) Don't start the blood-sugar rollercoaster. (3) Squeeze dry the liver glycogen sponge. (4) Don't feed the fermenting gut or the fermenting mouth with carbs.
Afternoon	No snacking. Quench your thirst with water. Black coffee or tea.	Squeeze dry the liver glycogen sponge.
Supper	Low GI foods.	Fill the liver and muscle glycogen metabolic sponges. (Though food is low GI, lack of physical or mental exercise, because we are tired, and the nightly fall in basal metabolic rate to promote sleep, mean there is surplus carbohydrate available to replenish the glycogen sponges.)
	High GI foods with or after the meal.	Slow the sugar rush to the liver so it does not overwhelm its ability to mop up. Rinse the mouth with water to wash off carbohydrates/sugars which stick to the teeth.
Evening	No snacking.	

Time	Action	Mechanism
Bedtime	Vitamin C to bowel tolerance.	Brush teeth with a neem toothpaste that does not contain sugar or fluoride. Zinc 30 milligrams reduces fermenting microbes in the upper gut. Neem is directly toxic to fermenting microbes in the mouth. Improves insulin sensitivity.
Once a week	Do not eat supper.	This really squeezes the liver metabolic sponge dry.
Alcohol	Use judiciously – just once or twice a week. Use a low-sugar drink, such as dry white wine.	Drink slowly preferably with or after food. This helps prevent the sugar/alcohol rush which switches on addiction.
Encourage fat burning	Find a pleasurable stress. Exercise, musical performances, entertainment, competition, sex, team-chasing of course, and being cold (ouch!) will pour out adrenaline.	Adrenaline switches on fat burning.

Conventional treatment of diabetes

Conventional treatment for diabetes is centred on prescription drugs, such as metformin, sulphonylureas and others (which increase sensitivity to insulin), with or without insulin injections, to bring levels of sugar in the blood down. The problem with all these treatments is that one risks dangerous hypoglycaemia (low blood sugar levels). To avoid this problem patients are advised to:

a) eat carbohydrates with every meal, including snacks. However, this compounds problems. The metabolic glycogen sponge in the liver can never squeeze dry. The fermenting mouth and upper gut are encouraged. This means that patients run their blood sugar levels high. This may be a short-term insurance policy against low blood sugar, but it has disastrous long-term effects for all the reasons detailed above. Furthermore,
b) no attention is given to the causes of insulin resistance (micronutrient deficiency or toxic blocking),
c) or to fat burning, though this is such an important tool to protect against the malign effects of hypoglycaemia.

In other words, the conventional treatment of diabetes does not effectively prevent (and/or reverse) the slippery-slope slide into chronic disease and premature death from damage to arteries, the brain, nerves, the heart, eyes and kidneys, and cancer. At best it slows this progression.

The upshot of all the above conventional treatments may be that the diabetes becomes 'brittle'. That is to say, it becomes increasingly difficult to stabilise blood sugar levels and the poor patient is constantly micromanaging through diet and timing of medication.

It is beyond the scope of this book to discuss the prescription drug treatment of diabetes, the indications for the various medications and the screening for long-term complications. This is beyond my experience and is the job of the diabetic clinics. However, it is my experience that if all the interventions I recommend are in place then it should be possible for type 2 diabetics to at least reduce and often stop their prescription medications and for the type 1 diabetics to need only minimal doses of insulin. In both cases, general health and life expectancy are substantially improved.

Chapter 7

'We cannot solve our problems with the same thinking we used when we created them.'

Internet Meme, wrongly attributed to Albert Einstein

How to lose weight

Once metabolic syndrome has been long established, a common result is obesity. We need to return to a normal weight for many reasons – not least of all vanity, self-esteem and well-being. As the old Irish joke goes, 'When asked the way to Dublin the traveller was told, "Well, I wouldn't be starting from here".' But here we are! Many people only start to recognise they have metabolic syndrome and/or diabetes when they are already overweight.

The key to losing weight is not to count calories and restrict food intake. This restriction of food intake will signal to the body that famine is here and so the body simply shuts down calorie burning to match calorie intake. If we stop spending energy (that is, if calorie burning is shut down), this renders us cold, fatigued and depressed. I have to say I am in awe of people who do manage to lose weight through self-induced famine and starvation – I know I do not have the will-power to survive such long-term deprivation.

To lose weight successfully, and keep it off for life, requires two steps.

Step 1: The first step is to put into place all the interventions to reverse diabetes and metabolic syndrome as detailed in this book. Interestingly, sometimes this is all that is needed to lose weight.

Step 2: The second step is to take advantage of 'metabolic inertia'. The idea here is that if we go one day with low calories or even zero calories, we continue to burn calories at the same rate during that day. So if, for the sake of argument, our normal intake is 2000 calories per day, then by eating 500 calories on a particular day this will mean that we will lose 1500 calories of weight.

The key to this diet is that we must go back to normal 2000 calorie per day food consumption the next day so that we continue to burn 2000 calories daily. If we do not, we gradually switch off calorie burning over the next few days and weight loss ceases.

We choose two days of 500 calories in every week (not consecutive days), hence this has been called the '5:2 diet'. The graph in Figure 4 shows how, when reducing calorie intake on Tuesday and Friday to 500 calories, the calorie burn remains at 2000 calories throughout the week, meaning that on those two days, 1500 calories of weight are lost.

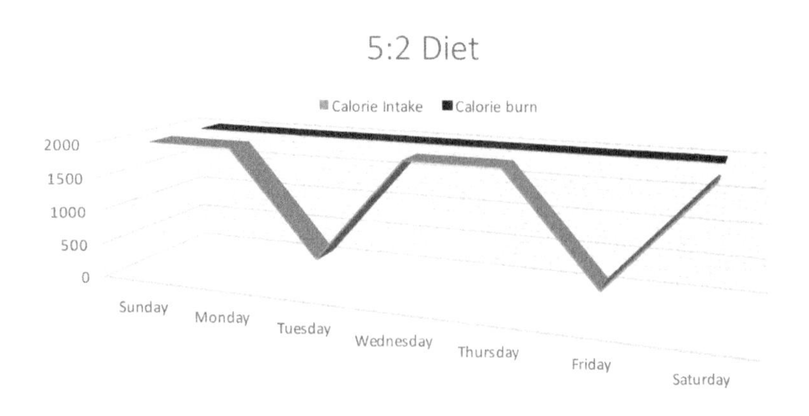

Figure 4: *Effect of '5:2 diet' on calorie burning*

Meanwhile, Figure 5 shows, schematically, the effect when a long-term reduction in calorie intake, say to 1000 calories daily, is undertaken. Gradually the calorie burn reduces to the now reduced calorie intake and at that point no further weight loss is experienced. The diagram is representative only and different people will take different lengths of time before their lowered calorie intake is matched by a lowered calorie burn.

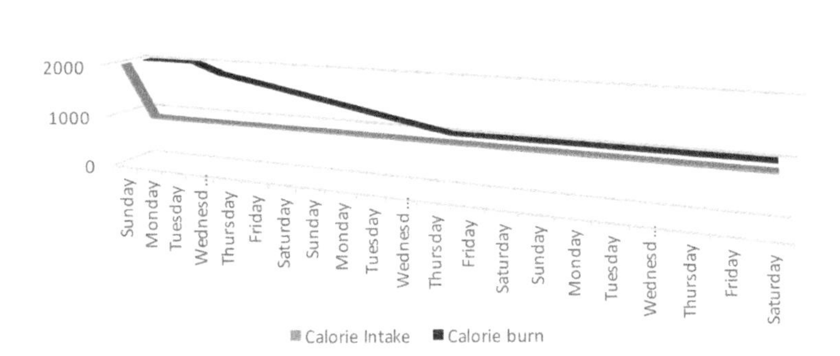

Figure 5: *The effect of long-term calorie reduction on calories burnt*

The ketogenic diet as a therapeutic tool

Metabolic syndrome and diabetes are the clinical pictures that arise as a result of fuelling our metabolism with sugar and starches. On the other hand, the ketogenic diet results in the body fuelling its metabolism from fats and vegetable fibre. What this means is that the ketogenic diet will protect us from, or reverse the progress of, any condition that is driven by metabolic syndrome.

It is biologically plausible, and indeed there are many scientific references and studies supporting its clinical effectiveness; table 14 lists those conditions that research has shown can be reversed and cured by the ketogenic diet.

Table 14: *Clinical benefits of the ketogenic diet*

Disease	Study details	Outcome	Reference
Diabetes	28 overweight type 2 diabetics on medication	21/28 completed the study. Medication discontinued or reduced in most participants. Fasting triglycerides decreased by 42%.	Yancy et al (2005)[27] www.biomedcentral.com/content/pdf/1743-7075-2-34.pdf
Diabetes	84 overweight volunteers with type 2 diabetes	49 completed the study. The lower the carbohydrate intake, the better the result. Medication discontinued or reduced.	Westman et al (2008)[28] www.biomedcentral.com/content/pdf/1743-7075-5-36.pdf
Heart disease	A comprehensive review of 36 medical papers	Ketogenic diet reverses indicators of heart disease – i.e. ketogenic diets improve heart disease risk factors	O'Hearn (2013)[29] www.ketotic.org/2013/09/the-ketogenic-diet-reverses-indicators.html
Cancer	Ketogenic diets recommended for the treatment of all cancers Ketogenic diet – review of its effect on 16 advanced cancer patients	They seem to be especially effective for malignant brain tumours. Pilot data suggest that a ketogenic diet is suitable for even advanced cancer patients.	British Society for Integrative Oncology[30] http://bsio.org.uk/ Schmidt et al (2008)[31] www.ncbi.nlm.gov/pmc/articles/PMC3157418

Disease	Study details	Outcome	Reference
Dementia	10 patients with Alzheimer's or similar severe cognitive impairment Low carb diet with fast 12 hours overnight. Nutritional supplements.	9/10 patients completed the study. All nine patients improved; six were able to return to work.	Bredesen (2014) [21] www.drmyhill.co.uk/drmyhill/images/0/07/Reversal-of-Cognitive-decline-Bredesen.pdf
Parkinson's disease	A comprehensive review of 55 published medical papers	'A growing body of literature suggests the ketogenic diet may be beneficial in certain neurodegenerative diseases, including …. Parkinson's disease…'.	Barañano and Harman (2008) [32] www.ncbi.nlm.nih.gov/pmc/articles/PMC2898565/
Inflammation	Ketogenic diet fed to animals for 14 days. Working with mice and human immune cells, these researchers focused on how macrophages — specialized immune cells that produce inflammation — respond when exposed to ketone bodies and whether that impacts the inflammasone complex.	Ketogenic diet exhibits anti-inflammatory properties. The results suggest that the endogenous metabolites like BHB that are produced during low-carb dieting, fasting, or high-intensity exercise can lower the NLRP3 inflammasome.	www.ncbi.nlm.nih.gov/ Peart KN (2015)[34] and Youm et al (2015)[35] http://medicine.yale.edu/news/article.aspx?id=8775 Dupuis et al (2015)[33] pubmed/26011473 NB – The inflammasome drives the inflammatory response in several disorders, including autoimmune diseases, type 2 diabetes, Alzheimer's disease, atherosclerosis, and autoinflammatory disorders.

Disease	Study details	Outcome	Reference
Infection	Review of 18 medical papers concerning the effect of a ketogenic diet on mitochondria and the subsequent effects of this A review of 16 cases of the treatment of urinary tract infections by ketogenic diet	A ketogenic diet not only rejuvenates, it also makes a person much less susceptible to viruses and bacterial infections.	'Every patient was in excellent health when discharged from the hospital.' Segura (2013)[36] www.drmyhill.co.uk/wiki/Ketogenic_diet_-_a_connection_between_mitochondria_and_diet Robb (1933)[37] www.ncbi.nlm.nih.gov/pmc/articles/PMC2369671/
Epilepsy	Comprehensive review of academic literature Ketogenic diet for treatment of epilepsy in children	'…there is growing evidence that the ketogenic diet alters the fundamental biochemistry of neurons in a manner that not only inhibits neuronal hyperexcitability but also induces a protective effect.' 'The ketogenic diet can be considered an option for children with intractable epilepsy.'	Kim & Rho (2008)[38] http://www.ncbi.nlm.nih.gov/pubmed/18301085 Rogovik & Goldman (2010)[39] www.ncbi.nlm.nih.gov/pmc/articles/PMC2902940/

Barañano and Hartman[32] conclude:

'The ketogenic diet is well established as therapy for intractable epilepsy. It should be considered first-line therapy in glucose transporter type 1 and pyruvate dehydrogenase deficiency. It should be considered early in the treatment of Dravet syndrome and myoclonic-astatic epilepsy (Doose syndrome).

'Initial studies indicate that the ketogenic diet appears effective

in other metabolic conditions, including phosphofructokinase deficiency and glycogenosis type V (McArdle disease). It appears to function in these disorders by providing an alternative fuel source. A growing body of literature suggests the ketogenic diet may be beneficial in certain neurodegenerative diseases, including Alzheimer's disease, Parkinson's disease, and amyotrophic lateral sclerosis. In these disorders, the ketogenic diet appears to be neuroprotective, promoting enhanced mitochondrial function and rescuing adenosine triphosphate production. Dietary therapy is a promising intervention for cancer, given that it may target the relative inefficiency of tumors in using ketone bodies as an alternative fuel source. The ketogenic diet also may have a role in improving outcomes in trauma and hypoxic injuries.'

The ketogenic diet to enhance athletic performance and treat chronic fatigue

I learned much about the ketogenic diet, keto-adaptation and metabolic inflexibility at a conference on mitochondrial function at the John Radcliffe Hospital in 2013. This conference was delivered by Professor Kieran Clarke (see www.dpag.ox.ac.uk/team/kieran-clarke). One paper that was presented at this conference was produced in response to problems that had arisen during the Gulf War. Frontline troops were told that they had to expect to function independently, without back-up, for five days, and, therefore, they had to carry with them all their needs to achieve this. Most troops chose to carry extra ammunition at the expense of carrying food. These troops were clearly carbohydrate addicts – after a few days they were not functioning normally and, indeed, most of the deaths from friendly fire occurred during the latter days from hypoglycaemic, non-keto-adapted troops making bad decisions. In the wake of this disaster, the United States army commissioned a study into what would constitute the lightest but most efficient food for troops to carry.

This food was found to be beta-hydroxybutyric acid; this is a ketone body produced when fats are mobilised as a fuel resource. It is difficult to manufacture outside the human body but a laboratory in Oxford managed to produce some. This was supplied in the form of a disgustingly flavoured drink at a dose of 1.5 grams of beta-hydroxybutyrate per kilogram of body weight per day. This drink was tested on elite athletes, who found that while they were on it they were not hungry. All lost weight (probably glycogen and water – see below). However, despite this weight loss their performance increased by 7%. From an elite athlete this is an astonishing improvement and would make the difference between an also-ran and a gold-medal performance.

We know already from the work of Drs Stephen Phinney and Jeff Volek that athletic performance can be enhanced by a ketogenic diet.[20] Dietary training is required to switch on fat burning, but once this has been achieved there are clear benefits.

1. The fat fuel tank has huge storage capacity compared with the sugar glycogen fuel tank. At best, the sugar glycogen fuel tank can store 2000 kCal. An elite athlete with just 10% body fat, once keto-adapted, has a fuel tank of 40,000 kCal. Our keto-adapted athlete can run much further.
2. There is also a power-weight benefit. One gram of glycogen delivers 4 kCal, but holds two grams of water. By contrast, one gram of fat generates 9 kCal of energy. So, for a carb addict to generate 500 kCal of energy he must carry 125 grams of glycogen and 250 grams of water, a total of 375 grams. Our keto-adapted athlete can generate 500 kCal of energy from just 55 grams of fat. So the fuel tank of the carbohydrate addict is nearly seven times heavier than the fuel tank of the keto-adapted athlete. Our keto-adapted athlete can run much lighter.

Chronic fatigue syndrome

I have learned so much about energy delivery mechanism to the body through my work with patients with CFS/ME. As I get older, and perhaps wiser, I find that the very basic things done very well achieve so much. The vital aspect of treating anyone with CFS has to do with diet. Now I routinely put patients on low-carbohydrate, Stone Age type (or paleo) diets. For many this is the most important, but also the most difficult, aspect of treatment. There is much more detail in my book *Chronic Fatigue Syndrome – it's mitochondria not hypochondria*.

Essential practical details for commencing a ketogenic diet

An overall guide for a ketogenic diet is:

- Protein content: 1 gram per 1 pound body weight – say, 150 grams
- Carbohydrates: up to 50 grams
- Calories: 2000 kCal (kilocalories) per day.

In order to achieve this, establish a list of very low-carbohydrate foods and make sure that your pantry is well stocked with such. Always look at the labels which detail the carbohydrate content of foods; this is very helpful. These carbohydrate values given on labels are normally total carbs, which include all starches, sugars and soluble fibre. Some people prefer to use net carbs (sugars and starches, with fibre excluded) on the grounds that soluble fibre is fermented into short-chain fatty acids. Linseed is a good example – it is said to have virtually zero carbs because, although 100 grams contains 29 grams of total carbs, 27 grams of this is fibre and so just two grams is starch and sugar. I find I can eat several slices of linseed bread and stay in ketosis, but some cannot.

Note that all carb amounts listed in Table 15 and in Appendix 12 (page 183) are given excluding the dietary fibre content.

By way of introduction, here is a generalised table of very low-carbohydrate content fats, oils and proteins:

Table 15: *Very low carb foods and amounts allowable in a ketogenic diet*

How much in a day?	...of which type of food? /Carb content	Important notes
Fat *ad lib* (as much as you like) (These are all saturated fats)	Lard, dripping, leaf fat, meat fat, coconut oil, palm oil. Carbs zero.	Possibly butter (but allergy to dairy is common). Saturated fats are the only fats that should be used hot for roasting, frying and grilling.
Oils *ad lib* (as much as you like) (these are mono- or poly-unsaturated)	Nut oil, seed oil, vegetable oil and fish oil. Carbs zero.	Only use these oils cold. (Heating them flips them to trans-fats). Make sure they are cold-pressed oils.
Protein (Approximately 1 gram per pound of body weight)	Meat (beef, lamb, pork, venison and other game) Poultry (chicken, duck, turkey, game birds) Fish Carbs zero *but* see next column...	...excess protein can be turned into carbohydrate by the liver. A ketogenic diet is *not* a high protein diet.

Other protein	Bacon, salami, sausage. Eggs. Coyo (coconut yoghurt – plain)	Very low carbs. There are 0.5 grams of carb in one egg. Coconut yoghurt (plain) contains 0.5 grams of carb in 100 grams, making it a great addition to the diet.

And here is a table of higher carb-content food types and the amounts of each that can be eaten in a day. (Note, the dietary data are mostly taken from the USDA [United States Department of Agriculture] Database Entry.)

Table 16: *Higher carb-content foods and amounts allowable in a ketogenic diet*

How much in a day?	...of which type of food? / Carb content in 100 grams is...	Amount allowed in a day to comply with recommended daily carb content (taken as 10 grams in all cases)
Vegetables and salad (Spiralised vegetables roasted in lard is a great dish)	Courgette 2.1 grams Green leafy vegetables (e.g. spinach, watercress) 1.4 grams Brassicas 2.6 grams Mushrooms 3.2 grams Green beans 3.6 grams Onions 7.3 grams Swede 6.7 grams Carrot 7.2 grams Butternut squash 10 grams Leeks 12.2 grams (**Note**: Take care with root vegetables) Potato 14.8 grams Parsnip 13.1 grams	**10-15 grams of carb** 470 grams of courgette OR 710 grams of leaves OR 380 grams of brassica OR 310 grams of mushrooms OR 270 grams of green beans OR 140 grams of onion OR 150 grams of swede OR 140 grams of carrot OR 100 grams of butternut squash OR 80 grams of leeks OR 67 grams of potato OR 76 grams of parsnip

How much in a day?	...of which type of food? / Carb content in 100 grams is...	Amount allowed in a day to comply with recommended daily carb content (taken as 10 grams in all cases)
Vegetables and salad	Lettuce, rocket 1.7 grams Radish 1.8 grams Cucumber 3.1 grams Tomato 2.7 grams Sauerkraut 1.4 grams Peppers 2.9 grams Spring onions 4.4 grams	588 grams of lettuce OR 555 grams of radish OR 320 grams of cucumber OR 370 grams of tomato OR 710 grams of sauerkraut OR 340 grams of peppers OR 230 grams of spring onions
Nuts and seeds	Brazils 4 grams Walnuts 7 grams Peanuts 7 grams Almonds 10 grams Linseed 2 grams Cashews 26.7 grams	**5-10 grams of carb** 250 grams of Brazils OR 140 grams of walnuts OR 140 grams of peanuts OR 100 grams of almonds OR 500 grams of linseed OR 37 grams of cashews
Fruits and berries	Olives 2.8 grams Strawberries 6 grams Avocado 2 grams Gooseberries 5.7 grams Raspberries 5 grams Blueberries 11.6 grams Blackcurrants 11 grams	**5-10 grams of carb** 350 grams of olives OR 167 grams of strawberries OR 500 grams of avocado OR 175 grams of gooseberries OR 200 grams of raspberries OR 86 grams of blueberries OR 90 grams of blackcurrants

The final table is of snacks and 'taste enhancers' which can be used to add variety to meals:

Table 17: *Snacks and 'taste enhancers' allowable as part of a ketogenic diet*

General food type	Specific examples	Important notes
Savouries zero or very low carb	Lemon juice Vinegar Garlic Mustard Salt Pepper Spices Mayonnaise and French dressing	None
Sweetener (zero carbs)	Stevia is safe and effective The sugar alcohol xylitol has a glycaemic index of 13 and so use sparingly. Both are antimicrobial.	Artificial sweeteners such as aspartame and saccharine are toxic. Other sugar alcohols (e.g. sorbitol, mannitol) increase glucose in the blood and are fermented in the gut.
Nibbles (zero carbs)	Pork scratchings	Once fully keto-adapted one should not need to snack – but eating crunchy food is satisfying!
Alcohol	Must be zero carb e.g. brandy, gin, whisky, vodka. The body 'burns' alcohol before fat – this may stall weight loss.	Care – alcohol tolerance is reduced on a ketogenic diet – you get drunk quicker. Will-power is reduced with alcohol. Don't fall off the wagon. Alcohol is toxic.

General food type	Specific examples	Important notes
Drinks (zero carbs)	Water or fizzy water Real coffee Tea Herbal tea (including green tea)	Always quench your thirst with water before drinking tea and coffee.
Chocolate (Gets its own section!) (say 14 grams carbs per 100 grams)	90% dark chocolate	70 grams daily equates to 10 grams of carbs *but* beware as too much may disturb sleep.

Dairy products: Most of the diets I advocate are dairy-free for the reasons I have given previously (see page 77). The safest dairy product is butter; it is the milk protein and milk sugar that are such a problem. Ghee is ideal since it is free of milk protein.

Have a go at some new recipes detailed in Appendix 1 (page 134). My life as a ketogenic was transformed by linseed bread, coconut cream, salad dressing, coconut chocolate, crumble topping and a spiraliser.

If in doubt, eat more fat and less carbohydrate.

You cannot rely simply on what you eat and how much you eat to know that you have done enough to get into ketosis. Some people can eat 100 grams of carbs per day and get into ketosis. Some have to reduce to below 30 grams (which includes me – damnit). Monitor your blood sugar and ketones using a Freestyle Optium meter. It takes about two weeks to become keto-adapted so do not be disheartened in the early stages. Women find it harder to get into ketosis than men, and we are all different. Measuring ketones in urine is not reliable *but* it may work for you. Ketostix for urine testing are less expensive than blood ketone measuring sticks. Breath testing is reliable, but the meters for this are expensive.

As you keto-adapt, blood sugars will come down and then they will become remarkably stable, fluctuating only by a few tenths of a millimole per litre. Ketones should appear and levels should be 0.5 to 3.0 millimoles. Levels tend to be lower in the morning and higher as the day goes on. After exercise, ketones may rise to 4 millimoles per litre. Please note, in diabetic ketoacidosis (see page 234) levels are above 10 millimoles.

There is a world of difference between the ketosis of low-carb eating and the ketosis of uncontrolled diabetes (see page 96). To compare the two is like comparing the thirst-quenching properties of water with water as a killer by drowning. Low-level ketosis is highly desirable metabolically speaking, but some doctors use diabetic ketosis – or keto-acidosis – to create a false alarm against the ketogenic diet.

Constipation may be a problem, in which case use linseed; this can be incorporated into the diet as linseed bread or as a crumble topping. As I have said before, although linseed has a total carb load of 29 grams per 100 grams, 90% of this is fibre and only 10% is starch. This means that some people can eat large amounts of linseed and remain in ketosis.

A ketogenic diet is demanding of minerals; you may need extra salt (at least two grams per day – that is, half a teaspoon added to food) and a good multi-mineral daily with 300 milligrams of magnesium.

Finally, remember that there are three major hormonal issues to be considered in order to get into ketosis:

1. A glucose spike (from a moment of indiscretion, such as snaffling a bar of cheap chocolate or a bag of crisps or a biscuit) will spike insulin and switch off fat burning for many hours. This means you will have a window of time of some hours when you cannot access fuel either from carbs (because the sugar spike has been pushed into fat by insulin) or from fat (because insulin blocks this). This may mean you feel awful for those hours. Knowing this is a good incentive to stay on the wagon.

2. To be able to burn fat you need thyroid hormones, so get your thyroid checked.
3. Female sex hormones induce a metabolic syndrome state.* This is why women have to eat fewer carbs than men to get into ketosis. I suspect the Pill and HRT have a similar effect.

Some people, especially if they are severely disabled, find that a ketogenic diet is difficult to follow purely because of the mental and physical effort of planning, preparing and cooking ketogenic meals. To this end, I have included Appendix 12: Ketogenic diet for the severely disabled and those with no time to cook (page 183), which contains, *inter alia*, seven days' worth of meal plans which require no cooking or food preparation, and also a shopping list which covers all of the foods that need to be bought to cover those seven days' worth of meals.

*Note: For the business of pregnancy and breast feeding, mothers need a store of fuel to guarantee their baby can survive. Female sex hormones achieve this by switching on metabolic syndrome which puts mothers into 'energy conservation, laying-down-fat mode'. Furthermore, during pregnancy, mothers run higher blood sugar levels than are usual so as to ensure that the growing baby is protected. This is because the growing baby is exquisitely sensitive to fuel delivery mechanisms and if sugar levels fall in maternal blood, serious damage to the baby results. So, female sex hormones, because they mimic the state of pregnancy, result in higher blood sugars being run, thereby inducing metabolic syndrome. Remember metabolic syndrome can be thought of as a loss of control over blood sugar levels. In addition, female sex hormones cause insulin resistance, leading to a further loss of control of blood sugar levels, and therefore, this further induces metabolic syndrome.

Chapter 8

How I persuade people to change lifestyle to reverse metabolic syndrome and diabetes

The big stick: Fear

There are times when I have to 'put the fear of God' into a patient, with all the facts I've covered throughout this book. I hate doing this – my job is not to terrify. However, I am more frightened of patients returning to me years later having had their stroke, or cancer, or heart disease diagnosis with an accusing look in their eye: 'Why didn't you tell me?' I prefer it when people frighten themselves. This happens either when they develop symptoms or when someone close to them succumbs and they are suddenly faced with the question, 'Why?'

A good friend of mine gave up smoking when I looked into the back of his eye and could see his arteries exhibiting 'silver wirings' – in other words, early hardening.

Fear of death and disease may work for some, but does not work for younger people, especially men, because of course they are immortal. I have to turn to the carrot.

The carrot: Vanity

> *'vanitas vanitatum omnia vanitas' – 'vanity of vanities; everything [is] vanity'*
>
> Vulgate Bible, *Ecclesiastes* 1:2; 12:8

The understanding that metabolic syndrome makes one 'ugly' and 'stupid', grow fat and have cellulite is often remarkably helpful. Indeed, it took the following incident to make me realise the power of vanity:

> The heavens opened, the rain poured, the river rose so the ford to access Upper Weston was flooded and impassable. My girls rejoiced because they could not get to school; patients had to be postponed. However, one patient, Rosemary, was desperate for an injection so I offered to do such by paddling across the river. I reckoned my best bet was to wear trainers and shorts to reduce the drag of the water and the chances of my being swept downstream. Suitably attired, I appeared in the kitchen to the complete horror of Ruth and Claire. I started to address their assumed concerns – of course they did not want Mother bowled over to a watery doom. I inwardly smiled at their love, pleased that they were thinking of my welfare. Wrong! It was not my welfare that they had in mind. 'No, no,' they said, 'You can't go like that – you haven't shaved your legs.'

I spend much more time persuading people that they must change than explaining how to change. The degree of resistance to change is directly proportionate to how addicted they are to their diet. The more reasons they give me not to change reflects this. The commonest Q and A scenarios are as follows:

Table 18: *The usual excuses for not changing lifestyle*

'I've always eaten like this.'	We can't solve problems by using the same kind of thinking we used when we created them.
'I have not got the time to change.'	In that case you are not ill enough or frightened enough.
'The Stone Age diet is boring.' 'Food is my reward at the end of a hard day's work.' 'Food is my main pleasure in life – this is a bereavement.'	These comments arise when people muddle the sensations of taste and addiction. What they mean is that they do not get a psychological hit after a meal if they give up the bad stuff.
'If I cut out grains, dairy and sugar, then there is nothing left for me to eat.'	There are over 20,000 edible plants in the world. None of my patients has yet starved to death.

Finally: Don't trust doctors

Patients are often under the misapprehension that their diabetes is being effectively treated because the doctors at their diabetic clinic pronounce satisfaction with their results. As detailed above, the goal posts for blood sugar are manipulated to protect against low blood sugar and so make life easy for doctors and patients alike, but this is short-term gain and long-term pain. The biochemical havoc remains and pathology progresses. How do I know this? Because much of standard medical treatment has to do with mopping up the mess of diseased arteries, hearts, brains, eyes and kidneys, and cancer. The cynic in me tells me this is a wonderful profit creation scheme for Big Pharma.

The first lesson that must be learned is that the patient is his best doctor – he has a powerful vested interest in sickness and in getting well. Do not rely on doctors – doctors are dangerous (see page 177).

Conclusion

This brings us to the end of our journey. For me it has been a rollercoaster ride driven by fear and addiction. I hope I have done enough to persuade you to change. I too am an addict and have every sympathy for those fighting short-term emotional comfort for long-term intellectual gain. I hope I have given you enough weapons to fight and win. It is a battle for life that we will all fight for life.

Perhaps true immortality is achieved as Horace put forward: '*non omnis moriar*' – 'not all of me shall die' – indicating that part of the orator, the writer, the artist, lives on in his work, after his death.

NOTE: Craig's father, Sqn Ldr Peter Bryan Robinson RAF Regt (Ret'd) BEM sadly passed away in 2014. Ever since Craig and his brother, Bryn, were young, they remember a three-word phrase that he would always repeat at difficult times. It is perhaps apposite to mention it here, as a final reminder to those who need one more gentle push into the difficult, yet worthwhile, challenge of changing their lifestyle and reaping the rewards: 'Nothing is impossible'.

Sqn Ldr Peter Bryan Robinson RAF Regt (Ret'd) BEM
(6 July 1926 to 11 October 2014)

References

Chapter 1: Introduction

1. Darwin C. *The Descent of Man, and Selection in Relation to Sex*. Page 12. http://darwin-online.org.uk/converted/published/1871_Descent_F937/1871_Descent_F937.1.html
2. Pauling L. As quoted by Francis Crick in his presentation *The Impact of Linus Pauling on Molecular Biology* (1995) https://en.wikiquote.org/wiki/Linus_Pauling

Chapter 2: Sugar – our non-essential and dangerous fuel

3. Reinwald H. Healing the glutoxic brain – and sugar and cancer. Presentation at BSEM Conference: Sugar... the Brain, the Microbiome and Cancer. October 2015. http://www.foodsmatter.com/conference_reports/articles/bsem-10-15-sugar.html
4. Teichholz N. The science of saturated fat: a big fat surprise about nutrition? *The Independent* 26 August 2014. http://www.independent.co.uk/life-style/health-and-families/features/the-science-of-saturated-fat-a-big-fat-surprise-about-nutrition-9692121.html
5. Malhotra A. Saturated fat is not the major issue – let's bust the myth of its role in heart disease. *BMJ* 2013; 347: f6340. doi: 10.1136/bmj.f6340 http://journals.bmj.com/site/bmj/statins/SP16c%20Malhotra%20October%202013%20with%20comments%20final%20from%20RC.pdf

6. Yudkin J, Lustig R. *Pure, White and Deadly: How sugar is killing us and what we can do to stop it.* Revised edition. UK: Penguin; 2012.
7. Finch CE. Herodotus on Diet and Longevity: How the Persians fed on dung and lived to 80, while the tall, handsome Ethiopians ate boiled meat and lived beyond 120. *Journal of Aging, Humanities, and the Arts* 2009; 3(2): 86-96. DOI: 10.1080/19325610902833247 http://www.tandfonline.com/doi/abs/10.1080/19325610902833247

Chapter 3: How sugar damages the body

8. Ritholtz B. *Bailout Nation – how greed and easy money corrupted Wall Street and shook the world economy.* US: John Wiley & Sons; 2010.
9. Monte M de la, Wands JR. Alzheimer's disease is type 3 diabetes – evidence reviewed. *Journal of Diabetes Science and Technology.* 2008; 2(6): 1101-1113.
   www.ncbi.nlm.nih.gov/pmc/articles/PMC2769828/
10. Dawkins R *The Selfish Gene* Oxford, UK: Oxford University Press; 1976.
11. O'Boyle CJ, MacFie J, Mitchell CJ, Johnstone D, Sagar PM, Sedman PC. Microbiology of bacterial translocation in humans. *Gut* 1998; 42(1): 29-35.
   www.ncbi.nlm.nih.gov/pubmed/9505882
12. Nishihara K. Disclosure of the major causes of mental illness – mitochondrial deterioration in brain neurons via opportunistic infection. *Journal of Biological Physics and Chemistry* 2012; 12: 11-18. DOI: 10.4024/38NI11A.jbpc.12.01
   http://inovanature.com/pdf/NISHIHARA.pdf

Chapter 4: Diagnosis of diabetes and metabolic disorder

13. Hyde D. The 10 most sugary breakfast cereals. *Daily Telegraph* 28 January 2015
   www.telegraph.co.uk/news/shopping-and-consumer-news/11373080/The-10-most-sugary-breakfast-cereals.html

Chapter 5: Why sugar and refined carbohydrates have become such a problem

14. Hansard: Royal Navy (rum ration). HC Deb 28 January 1970 vol 794 cc1660-86

http://hansard.millbanksystems.com/commons/1970/jan/28/royal-navy-rum-ration

15. Adamson A et al. *School Food Standards – a practical guide for schools, their cooks and caterers*. July 2013. Published by The Independent School Food Plan, financed by the Department of Education, Defra and Public Health England, the Rothschild Foundation, the Sainsburys Charitable Trusts, and other trusts. www.schoolfoodplan.com/wp-content/uploads/2015/01/School-Food-Standards-Guidance-FINAL-V3.pdf

Chapter 6: How the body controls levels of sugar in the bloodstream

16. Nordquist C. What happens during acute inflammation. *Medical News Today* updated 16 December 2015; accessed December 2015. www.medicalnewstoday.com/articles/248423.php?page=2
17. Pond C. Adipose tissue and the immune system. *Prostaglandins, Leukotrienes and Essential Fatty Acids* 2005; 73: 17-30. www.ncbi.nlm.nih.gov/pubmed/15946832
18. Lee DH, Lee IK, Song K, Toscano W, Baker BA, Jacobs DR Jr. A strong dose-response relation between serum concentrations of persistent organic pollutants and diabetes: results from the National Health and Examination Survey 1999-2002. *Diabetes Care* 2006; 29(7): 1638-1644. www.ncbi.nlm.nih.gov/pubmed/16801591
19. Porta M. Editorial: Persistent organic pollutants and the burden of diabetes. *Lancet* 2006; 368(9535): 558-559. www.ncbi.nlm.nih.gov/pubmed/16905002

Chapter 7 – Prevention, treatment and reversal of metabolic syndrome and diabetes

20. Westman E, Phinney S, Volek J. *New Atkins, New You*. US: Vermilion; 2010.
21. Bredesen DE. Reversal of cognitive decline – a novel therapeutic approach. *Aging* 2014; 6(9): 707-717. www.doctormyhill.co.uk/drmyhill/images/0/07/Reversal-of-Cognitive-decline-Bredesen.pdf
22. Toft A. *Understanding thyroid disorders*. London, UK: BMA (Family Doctor Publications Ltd); 2008.

23. Koulouri O, Moran C, Halsall D, Chatterjee K, Gurnell M. Pitfalls in the measurement and interpretation of thyroid function tests. *Best Practice & Research: Clinical Endocrinology & Metabolism* 2013; 27(6): 745–762. doi: 10.1016/j.beem.2013.10.003. www.ncbi.nlm.nih.gov/pubmed/24275187
24. Blanchard K & Abrams Brill M. *What Your Doctor May Not Tell You About Hypothyroidism.* US: Grand Central Publishing; 2004.
25. Robinson P. *Recovering with T3: my journey from hypothyroidism to good health using the T3 thyroid hormone.* US: Elephant in the Room Books; 2013.
26. Drenick EJ, Alavrez LC, Tamasi GC, Brickman AS. Resistance to symptomatic insulin reactions after fasting. *Journal of Clinical Investigation* 1972; 51(10): 2757–2762. doi: 10.1172/JCI107095 www.ncbi.nlm.nih.gov/pmc/articles/PMC332976/
27. Yancy WS Jr, Foy M, Allison M Chalecki AM, Vernon MC, Westman EC. A low-carbohydrate, ketogenic diet to treat type 2 diabetes. *Nutrition & Metabolism* 2005; 2:34 doi:10.1186/1743-7075-2-3 www.biomedcentral.com/content/pdf/1743-7075-2-34.pdf
28. Westman EC, Yancy WS Jr, Mavropoulos JC, Marquart M, McDuffie JR. The effect of a low-carbohydrate, ketogenic diet versus a low-glycemic index diet on glycemic control in type 2 diabetes mellitus. *Nutrition & Metabolism* 2008; 5: 36 doi:10.1186/1743-7075-5-36 www.biomedcentral.com/content/pdf/1743-7075-5-36.pdf
29. O'Hearn LA. The ketogenic diet reverses indicators of heart disease. www.ketotic.org (Posted 9 September 2013. Accessed November 2015) www.ketotic.org/2013/09/the-ketogenic-diet-reverses-indicators.html
30. British Society for Integrative Oncology. Website. (Accessed December 2015) http://bsio.org.uk
31. Schmidt M, Pfetzer N, Schwab M, Strauss I, Kämmerer U. Effects of a ketogenic diet on the quality of life in 16 patients with advanced cancer: A pilot trial. *Nutrition and Metabolism (London)* 2011; 8: 54. DOI: 10.1186/1743-7075-8-54 www.ncbi.nlm.nih.gov/pmc/articles/PMC3157418/
32. Barañano KW, Hartman AL. The Ketogenic Diet: Uses in Epilepsy and Other Neurologic Illnesses. *Current Treatment Options in Neurology* 2008; 10(6): 410-419. www.ncbi.nlm.nih.gov/pmc/articles/PMC2898565/
33. Dupuis N, Curatolo N, Benoist JF, Auvin S. Ketogenic diet exhibits anti-inflammatory properties. Epilepsia 2015; 56(7): e95-98. doi: 10.1111/epi.13038.

www.ncbi.nlm.nih.gov/pubmed/26011473
34. Peart KN. Anti-inflammatory mechanism of dieting and fasting revealed. *Yale News* 16 February 2015.
http://medicine.yale.edu/news/article.aspx?id=8775
35. Youm Y-H et al. The ketone metabolite beta-hydroxybutyrate blocks NLRP3 inflammasome-mediated inflammatory disease. *Nature Medicine* 2015; 21: 263-269. DOI:10.1038/nm.3804
36. Segura G. Ketogenic diet – a connection between mitochondria and diet.
www.doctormyhill.co.uk/wiki/Ketogenic_diet_-_a_connection_between_mitochondria_and_diet
37. Robb DC. The ketogenic diet in the treatment of infections of the urinary tract. *British Medical Journal* 1933; 2(3807): 1158-1162.
www.ncbi.nlm.nih.gov/pmc/articles/PMC2369671/
38. Kim do Y, Rho JM. The ketogenic diet and epilepsy. *Current Opinon in Clinical Nutrition and Metabolic Care* 2008; 11 (2): 113-120. doi: 10.1097/MCO.0b013e3282f44c06
www.ncbi.nlm.nih.gov/pubmed/18301085
39. Rogovik AL, Goldman RD. Ketogenic diet for treatment of epilepsy. *Canadian Family Physician* 2010; 56(6): 540-542.
www.ncbi.nlm.nih.gov/pmc/articles/PMC2902940/

Appendices

40. Ravera S, Panfoli I, Calzia D, Aluigi MG, Bianchini P, Diaspro A, Mancardi G, Morelli A. Evidence for aerobic ATP synthesis in isolated myelin vesicles. *The International Journal of Biochemistry & Cell Biology* 2009; 41: 1581–1591.
www.drmyhill.co.uk/drmyhill/images/7/78/Ravera_2009_-_myelin_makes_ATP.pdf
41. Dr Mary Newport. *Alzheimer's Disease: What If There Was a Cure?* USA: Basic Health Publications; 2011.
42. Pond C. Adipose tissue and the immune system. *Prostaglandins, Leukotrienes and Essential Fatty Acids* 2005; 73: 17-30.
www.ncbi.nlm.nih.gov/pubmed/15946832
43. Prynne M. Tooth decay is the biggest cause of primary school children being hospitalised. *Daily Telegraph* 13 July 2014.
www.telegraph.co.uk/news/health/news/10964323/Tooth-decay-is-the-biggest-cause-of-primary-school-children-being-hospitalised.html
44. Knapton S. Obese three year-old becomes youngest child diagnosed

with type 2 diabetes. *Daily Telegraph* 19 September 2015. www.msn.com/en-gb/health/medical/obese-three-year-old-becomes-youngest-child-diagnosed-with-type-2-diabetes/ar-AAeotMZ

45. Anonymous. The Thirty-Six Stratagems. https://en.wikipedia.org/wiki/Thirty-Six_Stratagems
46. Waldman A, Gilhar A, Duek L, Berdicevsky I. Incidence of Candida in psoriasis--a study on the fungal flora of psoriatic patients. *Mycoses* 2001; 44(3-4): 77-81. www.ncbi.nlm.nih.gov/pubmed/11413927
47. Nishihara K. Disclosure of the major causes of mental illness – mitochondrial deterioration in brain neurons via opportunistic infection. *Journal of Biological Physics and Chemistry* 2012; 12: 11-18. DOI: 10.4024/38NI11A.jbpc.12.01 http://inovanature.com/pdf/NISHIHARA.pdf
48. Albert HB, Sorensen JS, Christensen BS, Manniche C. Antibiotic treatment in patients with chronic low back pain and vertebral bone edema (Modic type 1 changes): a double-blind randomized clinical controlled trial of efficacy. *European Spine Journal* 2013; 22(4): 697-707. DOI: 10.1007/s00586-013-2675-y. www.ncbi.nlm.nih.gov/pubmed/23404353
49. Obituary: Dr Dick van Steenis – Campaigning GP who showed the link between air pollution and respiratory conditions. *The Times* 16 April 2013. www.thetimes.co.uk/tto/opinion/obituaries/article3739984.ece
50. Grant E. *The Bitter Pill: How safe is the perfect contraceptive?* US: Elm Tree Books; 1985.
51. Walesonline. Bovine TB research is 'flawed'. WalesOnline 3 Feb 2004. (Accessed January 2016) http://www.walesonline.co.uk/news/local-news/bovine-tb-research-is-flawed-2447887
52. Legler J, Fletcher T, Govarts E, Porta M, Blumberg B, Heindel JJ, Trasande L. Obesity, diabetes and associated costs of exposure to endocrine-disrupting chemicals in the European Union. *Journal of Clinical Endocrinology and Metabolism* 2015; 100(4): 1278-1288. doi: 10.1210/jc.2014-4326 www.ncbi.nlm.nih.gov/pubmed/25742518
53. Smerieri A, Testa C, Lazzeroni P, Nuti F, Grossi E, Cesari S, Montanini L, Latini G, Bernasconi S, Papini Am, Street ME. Di-(2-ethylhexyl) phthalate metabolites in urine show age-related changes and associations with adiposity and parameters of insulin sensitivity in childhood. *PLoS One* 2015; 10(20): e0117831.

www.ncbi.nlm.nih.gov/pubmed/25706863

54. James-Todd T, Stahlhut R, Meeker JD, Powell SG, Hauser R, Huang T, Rich-Edwards J. Urinary phthalate metabolite concentrations and diabetes among women in the National Health and Nutrition Examination Survey (NHANES) 2001-2008. *Environmental Health Perspectives* 2012; 120(9): 1307-1313. doi: 10.1289/ehp.1104717. www.ncbi.nlm.nih.gov/pubmed/18692848
55. Kelishadi R, Mirghaffari N, Poursafa P, Gidding SS. Lifestyle and environmental factors associated with inflammation, oxidative stress and insulin resistance in children. *Atherosclerosis* 2009; 203(1): 311-319. doi: 10.1016/j.atherosclerosis.2008.06.022. www.ncbi.nlm.nih.gov/pubmed/18692848
56. Thiering E, Cyrys J, Kratzsch J, Meisinger C, Hoffmann B, Berdel D, von Berg A, Koletzko S, Bauer CP, Heinrich J. Long-term exposure to traffic-related air pollution and insulin resistance in children: results from the GINIplus and LISAplus birth cohorts. *Diabetologia* 2013; 56(8): 1696-1704. doi: 10.1007/s00125-013-2925-x. www.ncbi.nlm.nih.gov/pubmed/23666166
57. Brook RD, Xu X, Bard RL, Dvonch JT, Morishita M, Kaciroti N, Sun Q, Harkema J, Rajagopalan S. Reduced metabolic insulin sensitivity following sub-acute exposures to low levels of ambient fine particle matter pollution. *Science of the Total Environment* 2013; 448: 66-71. DOI: 10.1016/j.scitotenv.2012.07.034. www.ncbi.nlm.nih.gov/pubmed/22901427
58. Suarez-Lopez JR, Lee DH, Porta M, Steffes MW, Jacobs DR Jr. Persistent organic pollutants in young adults and changes in glucose related metabolism over a 23-year follow-up. *Environmental Research* 2015; 137: 485-494. DOI: 10.1016/j.envres.2014.11.001 www.ncbi.nlm.nih.gov/pubmed/25706918
59. Lee DH, Steffes MW, Sjödin A, Jones RS, Needham LL, Jacobs DR Jr. Low dose organochlorine pesticides and polychlorinated biphenyls predict obesity, dyslipidemia, and insulin resistance among people free of diabetes. *PLoS One* 2011; 6(1): e15977. DOI: 10.1371/journal.pone.0015977. www.ncbi.nlm.nih.gov/pubmed/21298090
60. Burns JS, Williams PL, Korrick SA, Hauser R, Sergeyev O, Revich B, Lam T, Lee MM. Association between chlorinated pesticides in the serum of prepubertal Russian boys and longitudinal biomarkers of metabolic function. *American Journal of Epidemiology* 2014; 180(9): 909-919. DOI: 10.1093/aje/kwu212. www.ncbi.nlm.nih.gov/pubmed/25255811

61. Beydoun HA, Khanal S, Zonderman AB, Beydoun MA. Sex differences in the association of urinary bisphenol-A concentration with selected indices of glucose homeostasis among U.S. adults. *Annals of Epidemiology* 2014; 24(2): 90-97. DOI: 10.1016/j.annepidem.2013.07.014.
www.ncbi.nlm.nih.gov/pubmed/23954568
62. Wang T, Li M, Chen B, Xu M, Xu Y, Huang Y, Lu J, Chen Y, Wang W, Li X, Liu Y, Bi Y, Lai S, Ning G. Urinary bisphenol A (BPA) concentration associates with obesity and insulin resistance. *Journal of Clinical Endocrinology and Metabolism* 2012; 97(2): E223-227. DOI: 10.1210/jc.2011-1989
www.ncbi.nlm.nih.gov/pubmed/22090277
63. Khalil N, Ebert JR, Wang L, Belcher S, Lee M, Czerwinski SA, Kannan K. Bisphenol A and cardiometabolic risk factors in obese children. *Science of the Total Environment* 2014; 70-471: 726-732. DOI: 10.1016/j.scitotenv.2013.09.088
www.ncbi.nlm.nih.gov/pubmed/24184549
64. Howard S. *Diabetes and the Environment* website.
www.diabetesandenvironment.org
65. Lim S, Cho YM, Park KS, Lee HK. Persistent organic pollutants, mitochondrial dysfunction and metabolic syndrome. *Annals of the New York Academy of Science* 2010; 1201: 166-176. DOI: 10.1111/j.1749-6632.2010.05622.x.
www.ncbi.nlm.nih.gov/pubmed/20649553
66. Myhill S. *Diagnosis and Treatment of Chronic Fatigue Syndrome – it's mitochondria not hypochondria*. 2014: Hammersmith Books, UK.
67. Myhill S. *Sustainable Medicine*. 2015: Hammersmith Books, UK.
68. Starfield B. Commentary: Is US health really the best in the world? *Journal of the American Medical Association* 2000; 284 (4): 483-485.
www.jhsph.edu/research/centers-and-institutes/johns-hopkins-primary-care-policy-center/Publications_PDFs/A154.pdf
69. Diabetes UK. One million people in the UK unaware they have type 2 diabetes. Diabetes Health Intelligence at diabetes.org.uk. 30 June 2010 (Accessed December 2015)
www.diabetes.org.uk/About_us/News_Landing_Page/One-million-people-in-UK-unaware-they-have-Type-2-diabetes/
70. Grundy SM. Metabolic Syndrome Pandemic: Brief Reviews. *Arteriosclerosis, Thormobosis and Vascular Biology* 2008; 28: 629-636. DOI: 10.1161/ATVBAHA.107.151092
http://atvb.ahajournals.org/content/28/4/629.short
71. HSCIC (Health & Social Care Information Centre). National

Diabetes Audit Mortality Analysis 2011. UK: HSCIC; 2013. www.hscic.gov.uk/nda

72. Giovannucci E, Harlan DM, Archer MC, Bergenstal RM, Gapstur SM, Habel LA, Pollak M, Regensteiner JG, Yee D. Diabetes and Cancer: a concensus report. *Diabetes Care* 2010; 33(7): 1674-1685. DOI: 10.2337/dc10-0666 www.ncbi.nlm.nih.gov/pmc/articles/PMC2890380/
73. Pandey A, Forte V, Abdallah M, Alickaj A, Mahmud S, Asad S, McFarlane SI. Diabetes mellitus and the risk of cancer. *Minerva Endocrinology* 2011; 36(3): 187-209. www.ncbi.nlm.nih.gov/pubmed/22019750
74. Harding JL, Shaw JE, Peeters A, Guiver T, Davidson S, Magliano DJ. Mortality trends among people with type 1 and type 2 diabetes in Australia: 1997-2010. *Diabetes Care* 2014; 37(9): 2579-2586. DOI:10.2337/dc14-0096 www.ncbi.nlm.nih.gov/pubmed/24947787
75. NIH National Institute of Diabetes and Digestive and Kidney Diseases. Diabetes, Heart Disease and Stroke. August 2013. Accessed December 2015. www.niddk.nih.gov/health-information/health-topics/Diabetes/diabetes-heart-disease-stroke/Pages/index.aspx#connection
76. Emerging Risk Factors Collaboration. Diabetes mellitus, fasting blood glucose concentration, and risk of vascular disease: a collaborative meta-analysis of 102 prospective studies. *Lancet* 2010; 375(9733): 2215–2222. www.ncbi.nlm.nih.gov/pubmed/20609967
77. Jeerakathil T, Johnson JA, Simpson SH et al. Short-term risk for stroke is doubled in persons with newly treated Type 2 diabetes compared with persons without diabetes: a population based cohort study. *Stroke* 2007; 38 (6): 1739–1743. www.ncbi.nlm.nih.gov/pubmed/17478738
78. Strachan MWJ et al. (2011) Cognitive function, dementia and Type 2 diabetes mellitus in the elderly. *Nature Reviews Endocrinology* 2011; 7: 108-114. DOI:10.1038/nrendo.2010.22 www.nature.com/nrendo/journal/v7/n2/full/nrendo.2010.228.html
79. Holman N, Young RJ, Jeffcoate J. Variation in the recorded incidence of amputation of the lower limb in England. *Diabetologia* 2012; 55: 1919–1925. www.ncbi.nlm.nih.gov/pubmed/22398645
80. HSCIC (Health & Social Care Information Centre). National Diabetes Audit Mortality Analysis 2011/12. UK: HSCIC; 2013.

www.hscic.gov.uk/nda

81. Kohner E, Allwinkle J, Andrews J et al (1996). Saint Vincent and improving diabetes care: report of the Visual Handicap Group. *Diabetic Medicine* 1996; 13, suppl 4; s13–s26.
www.ncbi.nlm.nih.gov/pubmed/8894453
82. Arun CS, Ngugi N, Lovelock L et al. Effectiveness of screening and prevention of blindness due to diabetic retinopathy. *Diabetic Medicine* 2003; 20 (3): 186–190.
www.ncbi.nlm.nih.gov/pubmed/12675661
83. Glaucoma Research Foundation. Diabetes and Your Eyesight. Posted 18 May 2011. Accessed December 2015.
www.glaucoma.org/glaucoma/diabetes-and-your-eyesight.php
84. Gilg J, Rao A, Fogarty D. UK RRT Incidence in 2011: national and centre-specific analyses: UK Renal Registry 15th Annual Report: Chapter 1. UK: Renal Registry , 2012.
www.renalreg.org/wp-content/uploads/2014/09/Chapter_1.pdf
85. Shaw C et al. Comorbidities and Current Smoking Status amongst Patients starting Renal Replacement Therapy in England, Wales and Northern Ireland from 2009 to 2010: UK Renal Registry 14th Annual Report: Chapter 4. UK: Renal Registry, 2011.
www.renalreg.org/wp-content/uploads/2014/09/Chap04_Renal11_web.pdf
86. Shaw C et al. UK RRT Prevalence in 2011: national and centre-specific analyses: UK Renal Registry 15th Annual Report: Chapter 2. UK: Renal Registry, 2012.
www.renalreg.org/wp-content/uploads/2014/09/Chapter_2.pdf
87. Ziegler D. Diabetic Peripheral Neuropathy. In: Holt RIG, Cockram CS, Flyvbjerg A et al (ed.) *Textbook of Diabetes,* 4th edition. Oxford: Wiley-Blackwell; 2010.
88. HSCIC (Health & Social Care Information Centre). National Diabetes Audit Mortality Analysis 2011/12. Report 2: Complications and Mortality. UK: HSCIC; 2013.
www.hscic.gov.uk/nda
89. Diabetes UK. Good clinical practice guidelines for care home residents with diabetes. UK: Diabetes UK; 2010: Page 5.

Useful resources

Useful websites

Author's website
www.drmyhill.co.uk

Diabetes and the Environment
www.diabetesandenvironment.org

Thyroid UK
www.thyroid.org.uk

For access to tests

For all blood tests
www.bloodtestsdirect.co.uk

For comprehensive tests of nutritional and toxic status
www.biolab.co.uk

For comprehensive tests of gut function (stool) and hormone status (urine and saliva samples)
Genova at www.gdx.net/tests/search

Useful products

Accu-Chek mobile (for simple blood sugar checking on-the-go)
www.accu-chek.co.uk

Dexcom (for dynamic blood sugar monitoring)
www.dexcom.com

Multistix (for urine testing)
http://drmyhill.co.uk/wiki/Urine_MULTISTIX_analysis_interpretation

Freestyle Optium (for ongoing blood sugar monitoring)
https://abbottdiabetescare.ie/our-products/other-meters/freestyle-optium

Serious Pig salami
http://seriouspig.london/

Appendices

NOTE: All the following relate to reducing the risk of developing or maintaining diabetes and how to reduce that risk.

Appendix 1
Essential recipes

'The Cure is in the kitchen.'

Dr Sherry Rogers MD

For me, giving up dairy products and bread was a bereavement. However, I soon realised that part of my bereavement was missing the addictive hit which resulted from eating such foods. However, I have been able to find substitutes for these foods and my diet has been greatly enhanced by the recipes below, which are quick and easy. The following keep for weeks in the fridge:

Coconut cream
Coconut yoghurt
Chocolate cream
Coconut chocolate
Linseed bread
Crumble topping for berry pies
French dressing
Mayonnaise

NOTE: When I use the recipes below at home I mix metric measurements with Imperial. My publisher has insisted that both should be used consistently but I make no apology for the mixture. I blame Mother! There are many stories as to how the Imperial system, and, in particular, its reliance on the number 12, came about. We have

12 pennies in a shilling, 12 inches in a foot, and so on. One interesting theory is that we have 12 knuckles on our 4 fingers and these can be 'counted' with the thumb of the other hand. If you take the knuckles on, say, your left hand to count from one to 12 and the knuckles on your right hand to count as multiples of 12 (12, 24, 36 and so on), then using this system you can count right up to 144 (a gross!) using your two hands. Another historical point is that if you are stacking boxes, or such like, then a pile of four by three (12 boxes, say two by two on the ground and three high) is much more stable than a pile of five by two (only 10 boxes). In many ways, 12 is a more natural number for practical situations – it is easier quickly to find one sixth, one quarter or one third of things counted in 12s than it is for things counted in 10s.

Coconut cream

This is my favourite recipe. The resulting cream has the taste and texture of double cream.

Ingredients

one 450 ml tin of coconut milk

dollop of melted coconut oil (more for thick cream, less for thin cream)

½ teaspoon sunflower lecithin

stevia to sweeten, if required

Whizz up in a food processor and put in the fridge.

Use as you would cream – delicious in black coffee.

Coconut yoghurt

The same as for coconut cream but use fermented coconut milk.

Chocolate cream

The same as for coconut cream but stir in 60 grams (½ pot) Green and Black's cocoa powder.

Coconut chocolate

Ingredients
450-gram pot of coconut oil
125-gram pot of Green and Black's cocoa powder, or equivalent

Mix the whole of these two pots together and pour into ice cube containers.

Put these in the deep freeze.

Eat direct from the deep freeze.

Linseed bread

Ingredients
100 grams linseed ground up into a flour
20 grams ground almonds
½ teaspoon bicarbonate of soda
½ teaspoon salt
2 eggs
⅓ cup water
⅓ cup olive oil

Put the ground linseed and almonds, bicarb and salt together in a bowl.

Stir in the eggs, water and olive oil. Mix well or use a blender.

Bake in the oven at 150°C for one hour.

Slice thinly.

Crumble topping for berry pies

Ingredients
100 grams linseed ground up into a flour
100 grams desiccated coconut
1 teaspoon cinnamon
stevia to sweeten
dollop of coconut oil

Mix all the ingredients together, using as much coconut oil as is needed to stick them together.

French dressing

Ingredients
clove garlic, crushed
dollop olive oil
juice whole lemon
1 teaspoon mustard
generous pinch sea salt
pepper
½ teaspoon treacle, if you like

Mix all the ingredients together.

(The treacle is not essential, but it does blend with all the other ingredients to make a gorgeous texture.)

Mayonnaise

Ingredients
As for French dressing, plus
2 egg yolks
½ teaspoon sunflower lecithin

Whizz all the ingredients up together in a food processor.

NOTE: Get yourself a spiraliser. This increases the surface area of vegetables and salad so more fat, oil and French dressing can be taken up.

Cooking fat and scratchings

Purchase from the butcher leaf fat (the best-flavoured, lumpy stuff round the kidney and belly of a pig). My butcher asks me if I want it to feed the birds with. 'Yes,' I lie!

Cut it into grape-size lumps and put these into a saucepan.

Put on to a low heat – enough to melt the fat and sizzle slightly. Clear fat will run out and as it cooks, brown scratchings will appear in about 20 minutes.

Take these off with a slatted spoon, drain, add salt (unrefined) and devour!

The rendered lard should be white; if it goes brown then you have used too high a temperature. Use this for cooking – indeed I leave it in the pan and don't bother with the fridge because it keeps so well and I am constantly dipping into it, so it does not last long. Roast vegetables have never tasted so good.

Appendix 2
Why fats are so important to us

'Fat is the most valuable food known to Man'

John Yudkin (1910 to 1995)
Founding Professor of the Department of Nutrition at Queen Elizabeth College, London.

'... ye shall eat the fat of the land'

King James Bible, *Genesis, 45:18*

It has become so entrenched in the national (UK) psyche that fats are bad for us that I find myself spending as much time talking about how vital fats are as I do explaining how dangerous sugars and refined carbs are.

High-fat diets do not cause cholesterol problems

The medical profession, brain-washed by Big Pharma, has the cholesterol story upside down. The key factor is the proportion of 'friendly' HDL cholesterol. This is used up in the business of healing and repairing arteries (which typically have been damaged by sugar and high blood pressure). HDL should make up at least 20% of the total cholesterol. I have been collecting the cholesterol figures of my patients eating high-fat, low-carb,

Stone Age diets and the results are as shown in Table 19:

Table 19

Date of test	Gender	Year of birth	Total cholesterol (mmol/l)	HDL (mmol/l)	HDL/ TC %
Jan 2015	M	1938	4.4	1.8	44%
March 2015	F	1965	3.8	1.7	44%
March 2015	F	1935	6.5	3.1	48%
April 2015	M	1959	4.7	1.6	34%
April 2015	F	1963	6.4	2.71	42%
April 2015	M	1964	6.0	2.04	34%
June 2015	F	1974	4.7	2.7	57%
June 2015	F	1939	5.6	2.58	46%
June 2016	M	1977	4.0	1.6	40%
Juy 2016	M	1934	4.7	1.6	34%
July 2015	F	1975	5.7	2.5	44%
July 2015	F	1967	5.0	2.01	40%
July 2015	F	1953	5.6	2.6	46%
July 2015	M	1922	3.9	2.5	64%
July 2015	M	1968	6.2	2.2	35%
July 2015	F	1971	7.4	3.0	40%
Aug 2015	F	1953	4.4	2.2	50%

The high HDL percentages tell me that the arteries of these patients are not being damaged by high-fat diets.

Brain fuel

We know from work by Dr Silvia Ravera (Ravera et al, 2009) that energy delivery mechanisms to the brain are different from those to the rest of the body.[40] The vast majority of energy delivered to the body arrives as a result of aerobic respiration, which takes place in tiny structures in the cells called mitochondria; these are the little engines that burn sugar in the presence of oxygen to produce energy. However, in the brain there are not enough mitochondria to account for its energy usage; there must be another mechanism.

Ravera has demonstrated that much of the brain's energy is produced in the outer wrapping of the nerve fibres, known as the 'myelin sheath'; these sheaths are the fatty 'Swiss rolls' of membrane which are wrapped round each nerve fibre (axon) and deliver the necessary energy direct to that axon to allow electrical signals to pass. They have adopted mitochondrial biochemistry and are dependent on the fat they contain as a fuel, together with the oils needed to make the 'Swiss roll' membranes.

We know that if blood sugar levels fall too low, then the brain rapidly succumbs, loses consciousness and death may ensue. We also know from work by Dr Mary Newport that medium-chain fats, such as coconut oil, are highly effective in treating Alzheimer's disease, and the mechanism for this almost certainly has to do with improved energy delivery.[41] Therefore, we have good evidence, and furthermore this is biologically plausible, that the brain requires two fuel sources – namely, (1) sugar which is used by mitochondria where there are synapses (a synapse is the tiny gap between nerve cells across which one nerve cell communicates with another), in order to cross these, and (2) fat, to allow electrical signals to travel along a nerve cell's axon from one synapse to another. Low-fat diets are, I suspect, a major risk factor for dementia and this risk, I believe, is increased by the use of statins.

Immune system fuel

Work done by Professor Caroline Pond has shown that fat is preferentially deposited where the immune system is busy.[42] The immune system, like the brain, is greatly demanding of energy and it must have immediate access to an energy supply if it is to respond to the immune challenges of say, infection. Being underweight is a major risk factor for infectious disease because the immune system simply does not have the fuel it needs to fight the battle of infection. By contrast, sugar and carbohydrates fuel microbes and encourage their growth. High-carb, low-fat diets tip the scales in favour of microbes and infections because they simultaneously give the microbes more food and also reduce the body's access to the fat it needs to fight those microbes – a double whammy!

Storage of energy for hunting and survival

Fat is an extremely efficient way of storing fuel – weight for weight it can hold almost 10 times more potential energy than carbohydrate. For our mechanically minded readers, this is the difference between the steam engine and the diesel engine. This means that we do not have to eat as much fat (therefore, we can have a small gut) and we can carry fuel in an energy-dense way. This combination makes us an efficient hunter. Predators who power their bodies with fat do not have a large gut and, therefore, their power-to-weight ratio is good. Contrast this with prey animals which power their bodies from vegetable fibre – they have huge fermenting guts and so a poor power-to-weight ratio. The superior stamina of predators allows them to run down prey.

To be able to store energy as fat allows us to survive the winter when food is scarce. It also allows us to store up energy for procreation – pregnancy and breast feeding are greatly demanding of energy.

Insulation and shock absorbing

Having a good layer of subcutaneous fat allows us to live in cold climates. It even allows warm-blooded mammals like seals and whales to survive in freezing cold waters. Furthermore, fat is beautifully shock absorbing – our internal organs are delicate – in particular, the kidneys, and, of course, the brain. Fat is a perfect shock absorber and protects these organs from damage.

Skin quality

What gives skin its texture, water proofing and a barrier against infection is, amongst other things, fat. It amuses me that the product of our local meat rendering factory, lard, goes to the cosmetic industry – animal fat makes up a large proportion of cosmetic creams, lotions and ointments. Indeed, I suspect our current epidemics of dry skin, dry eyes, dry mouths and dry perineums may well relate to modern tendencies to eat a low-fat diet. Skin texture is a measure of beauty – which reflects evolutionary survival value. Fat in and under the skin demonstrates resistance to the common killers – cold, famine and infection.

Friction

Fat is an extremely important lubricant and allows tissues to slide over each other with minimal friction. I suspect modern epidemics of muscle stiffness and tendon and bursar inflammations may well relate to low-fat diets.

Appendix 3
Good fats and bad fats

Broadly speaking our bodies contain and use two types of fat: saturated, medium-chain fats and long-chain unsaturated fats. All fats are made up of fatty acids. It is the structure of these building blocks that determines a fat's character and potential usefulness.

The saturated medium-chain fats include lard, butter, coconut fat and chocolate fat – we use these as fuels to power the body. For the biochemists, in a saturated fat, every carbon atom is 'saturated' with either another carbon or a hydrogen atom. This renders the fat stiff and stable, so, when heated (which shakes things up), it retains its normal shape. These stiff fats are solid at room temperature.

Generally speaking, medium-chain fats contain between eight and 14 carbon atoms, whilst long-chain fats have more than 14 carbon atoms, and short-chain fats, fewer than eight. So, for example, approximately 50% of the fat content of coconut fat is made up of lauric acid (see Figure 6). Lauric acid has a melting point of 43.8°C and so is solid at room temperature. It has 12 carbon atoms and is therefore a medium-chain fat. In addition, it is saturated. Being a medium-chain saturated fat, it is therefore stiff and stable, retaining its normal shape when heated:

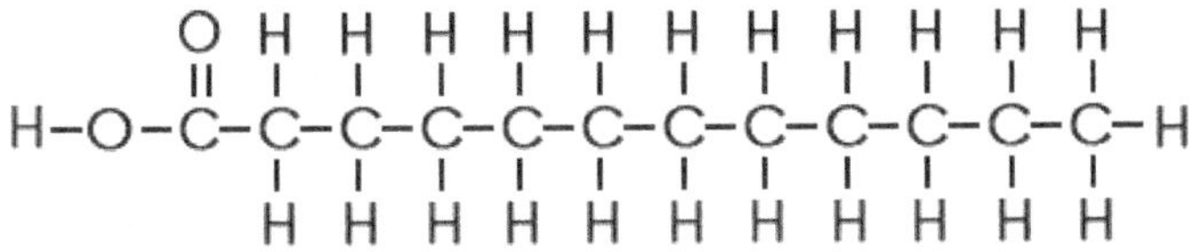

```
        O H H H H H H H H H H H
        ‖ | | | | | | | | | | |
H-O-C-C-C-C-C-C-C-C-C-C-C-C-H
          | | | | | | | | | | |
          H H H H H H H H H H H
```

Lauric Acid

Figure 6: *The structure of a typical saturated fat (lauric acid)*

The second type of fat is a long-chain unsaturated fat. The occasional hydrogen atom is 'missing' and so we get a double carbon bond instead. If we have one double carbon bond, then we call this fat 'mono-saturated' (such as olive oil) and if we have more than one double carbon bond, we call this fat 'poly-unsaturated' (most nut, seed, vegetable and fish oils). This double carbon bond 'kinks' the molecule and the molecule is named according to where it is kinked – such as omega-3, omega-6 or omega-9 depending on where the 'kink' occurs on the carbon chain.

Figure 7 shows how this 'kinking' may look.

saturated fatty acid

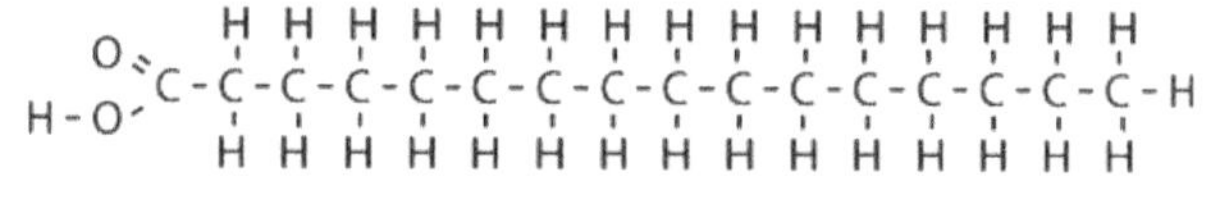

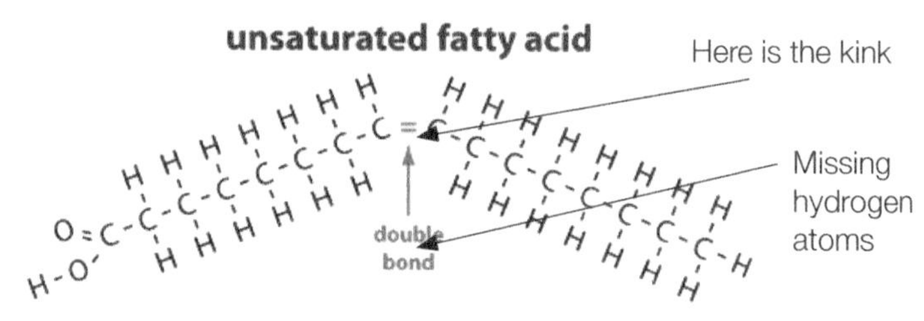

Figure 7: *The structure of a poly-unsaturated fatty acid compared with a saturated fat*

These fats are relatively flexible so are liquid at room temperature – we therefore call them 'oils' – and relatively unstable so they can be damaged by heat, for example, more easily than can saturated fats.

We use these fats as building materials – primarily for cell membranes. Indeed, many biological actions, such as energy generation and nerve conduction, take place on membranes. These fats are also called 'essential fatty acids' because the body can't synthesise these oils for itself – they have to be eaten.

In Nature, the kinks resulting from the double bonds are all 'left-handed' and are called cis-fats. They fit our biochemistry perfectly.

Problems arise when these fats are heated or hydrogenated (processed to render them solid at room temperature) and they flip into a 'right-handed' version; these are called trans-fats. Just as a right hand will not fit into a left-handed glove, so trans-fats do not fit our biochemistry, and so they clog up systems and are highly damaging.

Figure 8 shows the problem: the trans-fat is not the same shape as the cis-fat and so will not fit with our biochemistry.

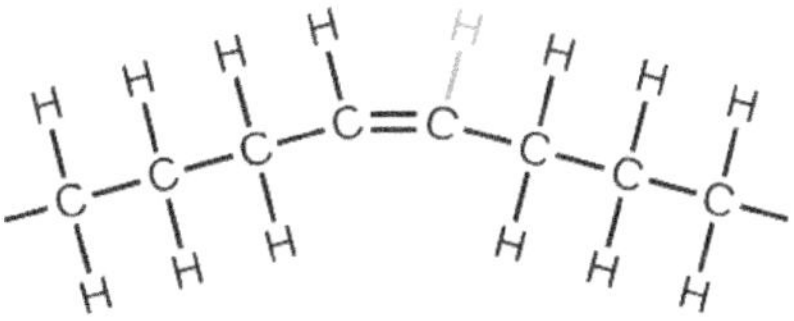

cis-**fat molecule**

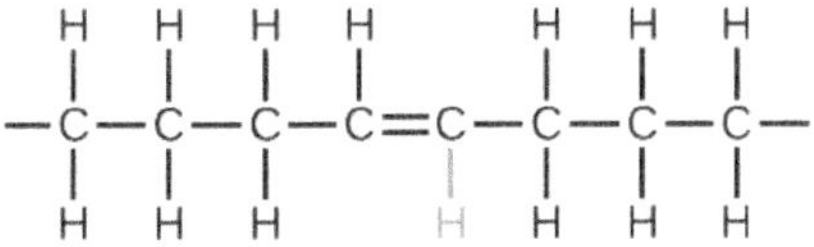

trans-**fat molecule**

Figure 8: *The crucial difference between a cis-fat and a trans-fat molecule*

The consequences of these factors are:

- Do not eat hydrogenated fats (as in margarine and 'spreads') – if the fat has been hydrogenated, then the resulting trans-fat will not fit with your biochemistry.
- Cook with saturated fats, such as lard (any animal fat), butter or coconut oil – these fats retain their shape through the cooking process.
- Use cold-pressed oils at room temperature – do not cook with them. Again, the cooking will heat these fats and so 'kinking' may result, meaning that these oils will not fit with our biochemistry.

Normal metabolism is so versatile that the amounts of fat consumed are not critical. General guidelines would be:

Saturated fats – Eat sufficient amounts to maintain weight and energy levels (mental and physical).

Oils – Only tiny amounts of essential fatty acids (EFAs) are required. They are called 'essential' because, like vitamins and minerals, the body cannot synthesise them itself; they have to be consumed. We all need omega-6 (linoleic acid) and omega-3 (alpha linolenic acid) EFAs in the proportion 4:1. These EFAs are present in all oils in varying proportions. I recommend hemp oil because it contains omega-6 to omega-3 in the correct proportion. I suggest a dessertspoonful daily – it is delicious and can be used in French dressings, mayonnaise or linseed bread (see page 134 for recipes).

In theory, these parent fats can make all other fatty acids downstream. However, in practice some people cannot do this and additional supplementation with other oils can have great benefit. I additionally recommend a fish oil supplement 1000 milligrams and evening primrose oil 500 milligrams.

Appendix 4
The fermenting mouth

Diabetes and metabolic syndrome occur side by side with rotten teeth because they have the same underlying causes. The fermenting mouth occurs when sugars and carbohydrates feed unfriendly microbes in the mouth. These microbes stick on to our teeth (we call this dental plaque) and punch holes in the enamel, rotting our teeth. They also attack our gums and it is indeed gum disease that is largely responsible for tooth loss. This rotting process extends into the roots of the teeth to form abscesses – the commonest cause of emergency hospital admission in Western hospitals for children is now rotting teeth requiring emergency extraction. Indeed, as reported in the *Daily Telegraph* in July 2014, figures for the UK showed that in the previous year 26,000 primary school children had been treated for tooth decay in hospital and nearly 500 children aged 5 to 9 years had been hospitalised for rotten teeth *each week*. In some cases, dentists had been forced to remove all 20 milk teeth because decay was so advanced.[43]

Rotten teeth kill us. Bacteria access the bloodstream directly, with the potential to cause infections at faraway sites, and this is, of course, further encouraged when levels of sugar in the bloodstream are high. Again, this provides microbes with a friendly environment in which to flourish. Diabetics are particularly at risk of these infections.

In parallel with the rise in hospital admissions for tooth extractions in children, we are now seeing 'adult-onset'diabetes in children. Sarah Knapton in the *Telegraph* reports that in the UK children have been being diagnosed with type 2 diabetes since 2000, with around 100 under-10s each year and cases as young as seven. In the US, which has consistently led the way on obesity, the youngest ever diagnosed is now a three-year-old girl in Texas, USA, weighting 35 kilos (5.5 stone), who was admitted to an obesity clinic suffering from extreme thirst and urination, the classic signs of the condition.[44]

Again, there is a two-pronged approach to preventing the fermenting mouth – do not feed the little wretches (the microbes, that is) and, secondly, kill them.

> NOTE: Here we are effectively using two of the famous '36 Stratagems' as advised to be used in politics and war, and as discussed in the Chinese essay of the same name.[45] These 36 Chinese proverbs are related to 36 battle scenarios in Chinese history, predominantly of the 'Warring States period' and also of the 'Three Kingdoms Period', perhaps from as long ago as 500 BC. So, 'starving the little wretches' is best exemplified by 'Besiege Wèi to rescue Zhào' stratagem , the meaning of which is, 'When the enemy is too strong to be attacked directly, then attack something he holds dear'. The thing the microbes hold dear here is carbohydrates and sugary food. And killing them is best exemplified, in this case, by the stratagem 'Kill with a borrowed sword'; our borrowed sword(s) are substances like neem (see below).

It is sugars and carbohydrates that are fermented in the mouth. As with the fermenting gut (see page 152), my view is that they should be permitted just once a day. This gives the mouth a chance to keep itself clean for the other 23 hours. Any sugars and carbs should be eaten at one meal, and after the meal the mouth should be well rinsed with water to wash away sugar and carbohydrate residues. An excellent toothpaste is Neem; neem is a plant that has good antimicrobial activity against the most pernicious of these fermenting microbes – namely, *Streptococcus mutans*. Indeed in India, neem twigs are used to clean the teeth after meals.

Of course, the body has its own mechanisms for keeping the teeth clean. Saliva is anti-microbial. How do I know this? Because in the wild, animals clean their wounds by licking them – this physically deprives the wound of soil and contaminations and in addition substances within saliva are directly antimicrobial. People with a dry mouth are particularly prone to tooth decay. The Romans knew this:

> *'Lingua canis dum lingit vulnus curat' or 'A dog's tongue, licking a wound, heals it.'*

As perhaps did Saint Magdalena de Pazzi who is said to have cured a nun of her sores and scabs in 1589 by licking her limbs!

You will know when you have done enough to prevent the fermenting mouth because your teeth should feel glassy smooth. Furthermore, there should be no gum disease or gum recession, no tendency to become 'long in the tooth'; trips to the dentist should be very occasional, simply for mechanical damage, and false teeth should become a thing of the past.

Finally, it is regular chewing of food that pulls our teeth and jaws into the correct shape. Modern diets high in carbohydrates and sugars are soft – children no longer have to chew – and this means they do not experience the correct physical forces which develop our dental arches, line up our teeth and improve our bite. As a result we are seeing epidemics of dental braces in children. We are once again back to the Great Masticator (see page 57)!

Appendix 5
The upper fermenting gut

The human gut is almost unique in the mammal world. The upper gut, consisting of the oesophagus, stomach and small intestine, should be a sterile, digesting gut to deal with meat and protein; the lower gut is a fermenting gut to deal with vegetable fibre. This combination has brought huge evolutionary advantages because it has allowed us to survive on a wider range of food than almost any other mammal (bar perhaps my favourite farm animal, the pig).

Problems occur when the upper gut starts to ferment foods instead of digesting them. This generates a toxic load which can overwhelm the defences of our fabulous liver. The 'fermenting gut' typically presents with symptoms of foggy brain and fatigue. Early symptoms of upper fermenting gut include wind, gas, burping, bloating, pain and reflux of stomach contents.

Farting is normal and occurs when friendly bacteroides ferment vegetable fibre in the lower gut to produce hydrogen and methane. These farts do not smell but they are flammable.

> I know this from experience. As a child my sister and I shared a freezing cold bedroom. If the frost appeared on the inside of the window we were allowed five minutes in front of the gas fire to get dressed. Our grateful bottoms would hover dangerously close

to the flame. On one occasion Tilly let rip and a sheet of blue flame leapt from the fire to the proffered pink cheeks, singeing the aforementioned. We collapsed with shrieks of laughter but the mirth had to be stifled as Mother appeared and we did not dare admit what had happened for fear of losing our hard-won morning glory. A stifled giggle is even harder to maintain and we nearly burst with the effort.

However, if we do not digest efficiently upstream, then undigested foods are fermented downstream to produce foul-smelling wind. We all do this if we over-eat and overwhelm our ability to digest. I have been doing this for nearly 60 years on Christmas day. I am reliably informed that eight pints of beer have a similar effect.

Professor Glenn Gibson, a food microbiologist from Reading, divides people into 'smellies' and 'inflammables' – normal gut fermentation produces hydrogen and methane which allows one to 'light one's own flatus', hence 'inflammables'. (Despite my sister surviving the incident above, I would not like to recommend this as a routine clinical test! However, this does mean that I am able to confirm that Tilly had a normal fermenting gut at the time of this incident.) Normal fermentation should be odourless. However, with sulphate-reducing bacteria present in the gut, hydrogen sulphide is produced giving the rotten eggs smell and a positive hydrogen sulphide in urine test. This situation ('smellies') indicates abnormal gut fermentation.

Conventional doctors clearly recognise the upper fermenting gut and call it 'small bowel bacterial overgrowth' or even '*Helicobacter pylori* infection', or sometimes 'SIBO', standing for 'small intestinal bacterial overgrowth'. However, there are many other microbes in addition to bacteria which can also cause fermentation, including yeasts and parasites. The fermenting gut, therefore, is a term which embraces all these mechanisms.

Largely speaking, it is carbohydrate foods that are fermented – that is to say, sugars, fruits, grains, root vegetables and other such. The body has to strike a difficult balance between taking advantage of these nutritious foods and not allowing fermentation.

A major line of defence against the upper fermenting gut is the combination of stomach acid, pancreatic enzymes and bile salts – all of these are toxic to microbes. Furthermore, they are an essential part of digesting foods, meaning that foods are rapidly digested and absorbed and so they are simply not available to be fermented.

Stomach acid is particularly important for three reasons:

1. It is a front-line defence against infection. Many infections get into the body through ingestion or inhalation – those inhaled get stuck onto sticky mucus in the nose and bronchi and that mucus is coughed up and swallowed. Microbes should find themselves in an acid bath which kills them.
2. An acid stomach is essential for starting the digestion of protein.
3. An acid stomach is essential for absorbing minerals and vitamin B12.

An understanding of these mechanisms gives us a clear idea of how we can prevent the fermenting gut. Indeed, as we age, digestion upstream becomes less efficient with two possible outcomes:

1. fermenting gut upstream and
2. the potential for undigested foods to ferment downstream and so the smellies begin to outnumber the inflammables!

In order of priority, preventative measures are:

1. Only eat carbohydrates once a day. I suspect it is the constant feeding of microbes in the upper gut, via carbohydrates at every meal, plus snacks and sweet drinks in between times, which allows these microbes to

thrive. Although the body does its best to keep the upper gut sterile by producing stomach acid, enzymes and bile salts, it is fighting a losing battle if we are feeding these microbes at the same time. Having a window of 23 hours a day when there are no carbohydrates in the stomach gives the body the best chance of keeping the upper gut sterile. (When I say sterile, I really mean low numbers of microbes because one can never eliminate every last one.)

2. Last thing at night, take 2-4 grams of vitamin C. Vitamin C kills all microbes. Furthermore, it is poorly absorbed and spends most of the night in the upper gut, thereby cleaning it up. It is humans, fruit bats and guinea pigs that cannot make their own vitamin C and we know that vitamin C is highly protective against cancer and arterial disease.

Symptoms of acidity should not be treated with acid blockers, such as proton-pump inhibitors (PPIs) or H2 blockers; not only do these prevent us from digesting our foods, but they also encourage fermentation, prevent us absorbing minerals and vitamin B12 and make us more susceptible to infections. As a result of these factors, acid blockers are a major risk for osteoporosis, degenerative disease, infections and, I suspect, all bowel tumours (oesophageal, stomach and large bowel).

There is much more discussion of the fermenting gut, irritable bowel, inflammatory bowel disease, acid reflux and treatment for such in my book *Sustainable Medicine*.

Appendix 6
The fermenting skin

High levels of sugar in the bloodstream have the potential to spill onto the skin where bacteria and yeast can ferment. This is an obvious risk factor for infection and, indeed, diabetes may present with recurrent boils, acne or fungal infections. These fungal infections include athlete's foot, ringworm, jock itch, fungal nails, dandruff, chronic vaginal thrush, balanitis (tip of the penis) and so on. Cradle cap and oral thrush seem to be pandemic in babies and again this reflects their, or their mothers', high-sugar diet.

Offensive sweat is another clinical sign to watch out for. Sweat is odourless. What makes it offensive is when it is fermented by microbes on the skin. Such fermentation is an evolutionary disadvantage – a hunter does not want to give his presence away to prey animals. Offensive sweat may be part of metabolic syndrome.

Eczema, urticaria and rosacea are allergic reactions which can be driven by allergy to microbes on the skin (and/or gut) – typically *Staphylococcus aureus*. I suspect this explains why the lesions of atopic eczema are typically in areas where the skin is thin.

Psoriasis, I suspect, is yeast driven – I am not sure of the mechanism but the connection is real, as has been shown by Waldman et al (2001).[46] As the authors say, 'Our results reinforce the hypothesis that *C. albicans* is one of the triggers to both exacerbation and persistence of psoriasis.'

Appendix 7
Chronic infection – life is an arms race

Introduction

You and I are a potential free lunch for bacteria, yeasts, viruses and other such parasites; indeed, we are a nutritious Petri dish on which microbes can and do flourish. There is a battle – an arms race – going on inside our bodies every second of the day. This is a race we can never hope to 'win', but only to stay sufficiently ahead of the game for as long as possible so that we stay feeling well. This arms race is a numbers game – our body must use its 'resources' to keep the numbers of the bad guys (the harmful microbes) down to a sufficiently low level so that we do indeed stay feeling well. That this constant battle is going on is clear – within minutes of death, when our bodies cease fighting this arms race, we rapidly decompose; the bad guys win and they win quickly. The business of fighting back against the microbes uses a great deal of energy – we know this too because if you give a normal person influenza, he/she immediately develops fatigue as the body diverts its reserves and 'resources' into fighting infection.

In my writing, and especially in my second book, *Sustainable Medicine,* I discuss the energy equation in detail. However, in brief, this equation can be very simply expressed as:

Energy levels = Energy Delivery *minus* Energy Demand

Fatigue is the subjective symptom experienced when energy demand exceeds energy delivery.

I have written in detail on my website and in *Sustainable Medicine* about how one can improve energy delivery (via interventions such as the mitochondrial supplement package) and also how one can reduce energy demand (via, for example, the use of EPD [enzyme-potentiated desensitisation], to reduce the immunological 'hole' in certain patients). Here we have another, and very common, example of an immunological hole in the 'energy bucket' – having a chronic infection. This hole is there all the time, causing a permanent drain on one's energy, and has the potential to become larger, if left untreated. The combined job of physician and patient is to reduce the size of this hole to an absolute minimum.

This 'hole' may well be the tipping point for some patients – that is to say, the chronic infection or microbial overload may push a particular patient's own individual energy equation into the red and make him/her feel really very ill. Likewise, dealing with this chronic infection and/or microbial overload may dramatically improve the patient's wellbeing.

I have talked about the 'resources' or reserves that the body has at its disposal to fight these chronic infections and/or microbial overloads. Here I have to consider what I will call the 'normal' state of affairs – that is, the way things have been in this arms race for the majority of our time on this planet – and then the 'abnormal' state of affairs – that is, the changes brought about in this arms race by the introduction of modern Western diets. The introduction of these modern Western diets has significantly tipped the balance of power in the favour of the bad guys.

These bad guys are a difficult enemy and persistence and patience are required to keep ahead in the arms race.

The normal state of affairs

We can never sterilise the body; we have to put up with a certain level of bacteria, yeasts, viruses and, sometimes, parasites. We have been doing this for millions of years – so much so that our DNA is at least 8% viral. We have done a deal with the virus – we will give it a comfortable home if it leaves us alone. This is the policy of pacifism! Trillions of microbes live in the gut. Indeed, if one totalled up all the cells in the body, including gut flora, then you and I are 90% bacteria. The strategy is twofold: both to keep the numbers of the bad guys down and to fill the gut with friendly, less demanding microbes (largely bacteria, but also some yeasts), which have an additional number of helpful functions, including:

- They have their own viruses, called phages, which kill unfriendly bacteria. Indeed, 15% of stool dry weight is made up of these bacterial viruses. Clearly there is a balanced predator-prey ecology within the gut. Predator-prey models are extensively studied within the discipline of Mathematical Ecology and Biology and generally there exist two of points of equilibrium – one where there are no predators and no prey (the death of both) and another where predator and prey co-exist in a steady state; this is the balance that we are looking for. For those who may be interested, please see https://en.wikipedia.org/wiki/Lotka%E2%80%93Volterra_equations and in particular look for the subsection 'population equilibrium'.
- They ferment foods to produce energy for the body. The most important of the friendly microbes for this function are the bacteroides. These are anaerobic bacteria in the large bowel which ferment vegetable fibre to short-chain fatty acids. These short-chain fatty acids nourish the lining of the bowel and, to a lesser extent, our bodies.
- They produce essential nutrients, such as vitamin K and biotin. These are essential because they cannot be

synthesised in the body.

- They help to programme the immune system. I have written about this extensively on my website and in addition, a new section on this will be included in the next edition of my book *Diagnosis and Treatment of Chronic Fatigue Syndrome – it's mitochondria not hypochondria*.
- There are probably other benefits of these organisms yet to be identified.

However, these friendly gut microbes are miniscule compared with human cells and all too easily spill over from the gut into the bloodstream and this can lead to very undesirable effects. We know both that these microbes do spill over from the gut and that they may cause undesirable effects from several pieces of evidence:

1. Ilya Metchnikoff (see the entry in Wikipedia – https://en.wikipedia.org/wiki/%C3%89lie_Metchnikoff), who first described probiotics and developed kefir, conducted an experiment where he drank kefir, collected his own urine and grew identical microbes from his urine. This indicated that these microbes had spilled over from the gut or they would not otherwise have been present in the urine.
2. Simply brushing one's teeth can cause bacteraemia (bacteria in the bloodstream); this is why dentists insist on antibiotics for patients with heart valve lesions prior to any dental work.
3. As mentioned in chapter 3, Nishihara has shown that fermenting microbes in the gut can be present in the brain with the potential to ferment neurotransmitters and cause psychiatric disease.[47]
4. Albert et al have shown the presence in joints of microbes which drive arthritis (hence arthritis can be cured with antibiotics).[48]
5. Interstitial cystitis, or allergic bladder, is a condition that I

believe results from allergy to gut flora and responds well to the treatment of such.

These are all, as I have said, very undesirable effects, but in the past the impact of these effects was not significant because of the diet that previous generations consumed.

The evolutionarily correct diet is zero carbohydrates (on a day-to-day basis) with an autumn bonanza of fruit and other natural harvests. This autumn bonanza temporarily switched on metabolic syndrome and weight gain and allowed us to survive the winter. We survived the winter on fat from fat reserves and fatty meat and fish. The important point about fat is that microbes cannot utilise it. How do I know this? I can leave a bottle of olive oil in my kitchen at room temperature for months and it does not go off. Ditto a lump of lard or butter in my fridge. Fat is what the body should run on. It is deposited where most work is done – notably the brain (which uses 20% of all the energy consumed in the body), the bone marrow (for blood creation), and round the gut (90% of the immune system is gut associated). Fat is an important defence against microbes because microbes cannot ferment fat. So fat is an important part of our longstanding defence against all the nasty effects I have noted above.

The abnormal state of affairs

We have a massive problem with Western diets because they are high in carbohydrates (grains, root vegetables, sugar, fruit sugar, pulses). These foodstuffs, unlike fats, are readily fermented by microbes. Given the right substrate, microbes can double their numbers every 20 minutes.

If the digestive tract is working perfectly, then these microbes are killed by stomach acid, pancreatic enzymes and bile salts. However, there are several factors which result in higher than acceptable numbers of microbes in the upper gut and put us at risk of a fermenting gut (see page 152):

1. Hypochlorhydria (lack of stomach acid) – caused by a leaky gut from allergy, infections (viral or food poisoning or *Helicobacter pylori*). There could be a genetic predisposition here. Once again, I have written about this extensively on my website and also in my books *Sustainable Medicine* and *Diagnosis and Treatment of Chronic Fatigue Syndrome – it's mitochondria not hypochondria*.
2. Poor energy delivery – so we cannot make the acid or enzymes necessary for normal gut function. This is a central issue in CFS/ME.
3. Nutritional deficiencies – so the body does not have the raw materials for normal gut function.
4. Ageing – as we age all the above factors come into play; indeed, we know this as most older people will tell me that they can no longer eat large meals because it overwhelms their ability to digest; they ferment instead and this is uncomfortable.

So, the combination of the gut not working properly (and therefore not killing the microbes) and the Western diet (too high in carbohydrates, leading to fermentation by microbes) leads to a problem with microbes both inside and outside the gut. Before I describe how to deal with the twin problems of microbes inside and outside the gut, we should first look at the symptoms which would lead the physician to the conclusion that the patient is suffering from a chronic infection and/or a microbe overload.

The clinical picture of chronic infection and microbial overload

A person with chronic infection presents with all the symptoms of immune activation as the body tries to reduce the numbers of microbes. These include the following general and local symptoms.

General symptoms

- Fatigue – This is an essential symptom to enforce rest so that the immune system has the energy available to fight.
- Malaise.
- Fever – Most microbes are killed by heat.

Local symptoms

- Mucus and catarrh – These physically wash out microbes.
- Runny eyes – Ditto.
- Cough and sneeze – These physically blast out microbes in the airways.
- Airways narrowing, wheeze, asthma – These result in the air we breathe becoming more turbulent so microbes are thrown against and stick to the mucous lining of the airways to be coughed up and swallowed.
- Vomiting – This is an essential defence against food poisoning and inhaled microbes (which are coughed up and swallowed).
- Diarrhoea – Ditto.
- Colic – Ditto.
- Cystitis – Emptying the bladder of urine means also emptying it of microbes.

Now, we can consider the twin problems of microbes inside the gut and microbes outside the gut, and how to deal with them.

How to reduce the work of the immune system

Reduce microbes in the gut

We reduce the work of the immune system by reducing the numbers of (bad) microbes that the immune system has to deal with and also by encouraging the friendly ones. This is a two-pronged approach – firstly, starve the little wretches out and, secondly, kill them. This means putting in place all the treatments to tackle the upper fermenting gut (see Appendix 5, page 152). I have also written about this extensively on my website and in my books *Sustainable Medicine* and *Diagnosis and Treatment of Chronic Fatigue Syndrome – it's mitochondria not hypochondria*. But, the most important treatment is the ketogenic diet.

Reduce microbes that are outside the gut but inside the body

This is more difficult because the body needs some sugar in the bloodstream to function and microbes can happily ferment this. These are not at sufficient levels to cause overt infection, such as septicaemia or abscess, but are present in sufficient numbers to drive a destructive low-grade inflammation. I think of this as microbial allergy. We need other methods to kill these microbes. Established options and suggestions are as follows:

1. Antibiotics, antifungals, antivirals – These are of proven benefit but resistant strains may emerge and side effects are possible.
2. Intravenous vitamin C (but this can be difficult to administer and is expensive).
3. Heat (pyrotherapy) – Sauna regimes are of proven benefit, but this therapy is often not tolerated in severe CFS/ME.
4. Light therapy – I have written about this extensively on my website. Please see www.doctormyhill.co.uk/wiki/Chronic_infection_%E2%80%93_Life_is_an_arms_race_%E2%80%93_how_to_tackle_with_natural_remedies#Light_Therapy

Appendix 8
The toxic causes of insulin resistance

For years I have been doing tests of toxicity with Biolab and Acumen laboratories, using blood tests, urine tests, fat biopsies and other such. Most of the chemicals being tested for come from inside the home – from furniture and carpets, cleaning chemicals and cosmetics. Indeed, I take this as a jolly good reason not to be house proud.

'My idea of housework is to sweep the room with a glance.'
Internet Meme attributed to Erma Bombeck

Below is a check list of chemicals to be aware of. As common things are common, the chemicals are listed in order of how often they come up in toxicity tests:

- Dichlorobenzenes – used in soft furnishings as insect/moth repellents
- Polybrominated biphenyls – flame retardants in soft furnishings
- Plasticisers, such as bisphenol A – used in food packaging
- Hair dyes
- Triclosan – a disinfectant and cleaning agent
- Solvents – in paints, printing inks
- Malondialdehyde – a toxin formed within the body that results if one has poor antioxidant status (lack of vitamins and minerals)

- Mercury – from dental amalgam and vaccinations
- Lead – from old water-pipes etc
- Aluminium – from baking foil, old-fashioned saucepans, foil packaging
- Cadmium – from cigarette smoke
- Nickel – often present in jewellery, so from piercings especially.

There are also toxins which I suspect are major problems but which often do not show up on testing – in particular, fluoride, silicones, glyphosate (the commonest pesticide), noxious gases (carbon monoxide, ozone, nitrous oxides) and products of the upper fermenting gut.

Prescription drugs can also be an issue – all those listed below increase the risk of diabetes:

- The Pill and HRT
- Statins
- Beta blockers
- Thiazide diuretics
- Steroids
- Anti-psychotic agents
- Immuno-suppressive drugs
- Protease inhibitors (such as drugs for HIV).

Toxic metals:

- Mercury – from dental amalgam and vaccinations, as above
- Cadmium – from cigarette smoke, as above
- Lead, as above
- Nickel – often present in jewellery, as above
- Arsenic
- Organotins (anti-fouling boat paint) – these are chemical compounds based on tin with hydrocarbon substituents.

Persistent organic pollutants (POPs):

- Dioxins
- Phthalates – a group of chemicals used to soften and increase the flexibility of plastic and vinyl
- Bisphenol A (plastics), as above
- Flame retardants – in soft furnishings
- Solvents.

Radiation:

- Windscale (1957) (re-named 'Sellafield'), Chernobyl (1986), Fukushima (2011) – all released radioactive iodine.
- A combination of all the above – air pollution from industry. A dear friend of mine, the late Dr Dick van Steenis, campaigned tirelessly to raise awareness of the disease-producing effects of polluting industry. Many of the above toxins are emitted and are a particular problem because of their size. Small particulate matter, which is invisible to the naked eye, is too small to be filtered out in the upper airway and passes straight into the lungs from which it is readily absorbed into the bloodstream. An obituary of Dr van Steenis was published in *The Times* in 2013.[49]

There are three people whose combined works have done more for the health of the nation than any other doctors I know. First there is the aforementioned Dr Van Steenis. Second, we have Dr Ellen Grant who has tirelessly flagged up the dangers of the Pill and HRT – she has hundreds of publications in mainstream medical journals and I do recommend her book, *The Bitter Pill: How Safe is the Perfect Contraceptive?* The Pill and HRT are so dangerous because they encourage metabolic syndrome.[50] Finally, we have Colonel Danny Goodwin Jones whose work correcting trace elements in soil has massive implications for the health of farm animals and humans alike.[51]

There has been a very large range of studies which have linked certain chemicals to insulin resistance. There is, for example, very convincing evidence from studies to do with phthalates and air pollutants.

- Phthalates – Legler et al (2015) conducted a European-wide study and concluded that phthalate exposure had a 40 to 69% probability of causing 20,500 new-onset cases of diabetes in older women, with €607 million in associated costs.[52] A further paper (Smerieri et al, 2015) showed increased insulin sensitivity among children with higher phthalate metabolites in their urine.[53] And, finally, for illustrative purposes, a large study (by James-Todd et al, 2012) of 2350 women over the years 2001 to 2008, within the National Health and Nutrition Examination Survey, concluded that: 'Urinary levels of several phthalates were associated with prevalent diabetes.'[54]
- Air pollutants – A study by Kelishadi et al (2009) of 374 children, aged 10-18, found links between exposure to air pollutants and insulin resistance,[55] and this is supported by a German study (Thiering et al, 2013) of 397 children, aged 10, which arrived at similar conclusions.[56] Finally, and perhaps most telling, researchers in Michigan (Brook et al, 2013) brought 25 healthy adult volunteers from a rural environment into an urban environment for a period of five consecutive days only and found that exposure to air pollutants was associated with increased insulin resistance.[57]

However, the story does not end there. There is also convincing evidence for a link between both persistent organic pollutants (POPs) and bisphenol A and insulin resistance:

- POPs – A 23-year follow-up study by Suarez-Lopez et al (published in 2015), in a sample of 180 persons, concluded that glucose-related metabolism was adversely affected in the age ranges above 40 years of age and this was only at background levels of POPs. In the age range 48-55, this finding was significant at a p value (probability) of 0.001 (meaning there is only a 1/1000 probability of this happening as a result of chance), making it statistically highly significant.[58] Another 20-year-long study, by Lee et al (2011) found links between simultaneous exposure to various POPs in the general population and the development of insulin resistance.[59] Furthermore, a study of 499 Russian 8-9 year old boys (by Burns et al, 2014), worryingly found that childhood exposure to organochlorine pesticides resulted in higher insulin resistance at 95% confidence levels, which is to say that we can be 95% confident that the higher insulin resistance rates among Russian 8-9 year olds are due to childhood exposure to organochlorine pesticides as opposed to random variation.[60]

- Bisphenol A ('BPA') – Beydoun et al (2014) studied 1586 participants from the 2005 to 2008 National Health and Nutrition Examination Surveys and concluded a positive association between BPA exposure and insulin resistance.[61] This was supported by a Chinese study (Wang et al, 2012), of middle-aged participants, which showed associations at the 95% confidence level, as explained above.[62] Perhaps even more disturbing, a study of 39 children in Ohio, conducted by Khalil et al (2014) concluded that higher BPA levels were associated with insulin resistance and various other metabolic differences.[63]

There is an excellent website resource, with much discussion and many more links to studies and papers, called *Diabetes and the Environment* (www.diabetesandenvironment.org) and this is recommended reading for the interested reader.[64]

Finally, there is a broader paper, 'Persistent organic pollutants, mitochondrial dysfunction, and metabolic syndrome' (by Lim et al, 2010) which concludes that environmental chemicals, including BPA, POPs and heavy metals, affect the functioning of mitochondria and thereby induce insulin resistance.[65] This links well with my main area of expertise, being the adverse health impacts of mitochondrial dysfunction, something which I have observed clinically as resulting from such chemical exposures. Indeed, increasingly we are seeing links between diabetes and mitochondrial dysfunction. This latter subject is another special area of interest of mine and much more detail can be found in my first, award-winning book, *Diagnosis and Treatment of Chronic Fatigue Syndrome – it's mitochondria not hypochondria*.[66]

Appendix 9
Tests – How to access tests to further investigate metabolic syndrome and diabetes

There are two aspects of modern medicine that I particularly dislike – firstly, the systematic obfuscation of causes of disease, and, secondly, the control of access to medical tests. The idea of this book is to empower patients with the knowledge and tools to take charge of their own medical problems. This section shows you how to access all the necessary tests to diagnose and start to reverse metabolic syndrome and diabetes. Of course, long-established diabetes may well need hypoglycaemic drugs and insulin in addition, but attention to the information below will greatly enhance the effectiveness of such interventions in those cases where pharmaceutical drugs are needed.

Blood sugar monitoring

Blood sugar monitoring is the single most important tool you need. The ideal is continuous blood sugar monitoring, such as Dexcom (see page 132) – but this is expensive. I recommend purchasing Accu-Chek Mobile (no – sadly I do not have shares in this company nor generously stuffed brown paper envelopes). Blood sugar can be measured in seconds and is painless (yes – I, too, am a wimp; I do not recommend anything that I cannot do). Note that it is important to wash your hands before doing the test simply because tiny traces of sugar on the skin will distort the result. Indeed, I gave myself a terrible fright when a blood sugar reading came up at 11 mmol/l. This was due to skin contamination with DMSO – a wetting agent to enhance transdermal absorption of magnesium. (No – DMSO does not affect blood sugar levels.) One hand wash and seconds later I recorded 5.3 mmol/l.

Initially measure blood sugar very regularly to see how high or low your blood sugar runs, but also to get an idea of the rate of change. With experience you will quickly work out which foods you can or cannot get away with. Remember, however – only one carbohydrate-containing meal a day.

Although the normal range of blood sugar is said to be 4.0 to 7.8 mmol/l, my view is that if the blood sugar spikes above 7 mmol/l then you are starting to lose control and so have early metabolic syndrome. Fasting blood sugar, levels after exercise and readings some hours after food should be between 4 and 6 mmol/l.

Stress will raise blood sugar levels; people often find that levels whilst at work are higher than at weekends or during holidays. This gives us just one more mechanism by which excessive stress shortens life.

Ketones in the blood

Ketones in the blood can be measured at home with Freestyle Optium. This is a really useful tool for demonstrating metabolic flexibility and keto-adaptation. Once the body has reached this state easily, not only does this greatly improve stamina and protect against the symptoms of hypoglycaemia, but it means one is greatly protected against metabolic syndrome, metabolic havoc and all its complications. Expect the following results:

	Ketone levels in mmol/l
Moderate carb non-fasting diet	<0.1
Moderate carb diet fasting and/or exercise	0.1–0.3
Very low carb <50 grams and/or exercise	0.5-3.0
Fasting	5.0—8.0
Ketoacidosis (type 1 diabetes)	10-25 – Not desirable – a hospital emergency!

Micronutrient status

I never bother to do tests of vitamins, minerals and essential fatty acids in someone who is eating a Western diet and not taking supplements because I know what the result is going to be – deficiency. This makes the testing at this stage a waste of money. We should all be taking a basic package of multivitamins, minerals, essential fatty acids, vitamin C and D. Once established on these supplements *and* the recommended diet, if blood sugar levels are still awry then further tests are indicated.

Nutritional checks

For these nutritional checks, if indicated as above, I recommend using Biolab. In order of priority I would recommend:

- Plasma and red cell elements (includes chromium, magnesium and zinc)
- B vitamins
- Vitamin D
- Anti-oxidant profile
- Iodine/creatinine ratio (urine)
- Vitamin C
- Essential fatty acids – erythrocytes.

All these tests can be accessed through my website, www.drmyhill.co.uk.

Thyroid function tests

These can be done on a DIY finger-drop sample of blood. Standard NHS testing of thyroid function is inadequate because it often solely relies on a TSH level. The bare minimum of testing should be:

- TSH
- Free T4
- Free T3.

The clinical information (signs and symptoms) is as vital as the biochemistry. So, for example, ongoing metabolic syndrome, especially if accompanied by fatigue, that has not corrected itself with the above diet and micronutrients, could well be due to borderline hypothyroidism. For much more information see my book *Diagnosis and Treatment of Chronic Fatigue Syndrome - it's mitochondria not hypochondria*.[66]

All these tests can be accessed through my website (www.drmyhill.co.uk).

Adrenal stress test

The adrenal stress test can be done on saliva samples and again accessed through my website.

This test measures levels of cortisol and DHEA in saliva in four specimens taken over 24 hours.

If levels of these hormones are high, this indicates a state of chronic stress. The treatment for this is to identify the cause of that stress up-stream, so to speak. This stress is commonly metabolic syndrome! However, any stress can result in this biochemical picture, be it psychological, emotional, financial, infectious or physical, or lack of sleep.

If levels of cortisol and DHEA are consistently low, this points to adrenal fatigue. As we age the adrenal glands become fatigued, but this is likely to occur sooner and to a greater extent if constant low-level stress puts ongoing pressure on the adrenals. As a treatment, a useful all-rounder is pregnenolone (also dubbed the 'memory hormone'). The production of the adrenal hormones starts with cholesterol, and pregnenolone is the first biochemical step. Cortisol, DHEA, mineralocorticoids and sex hormones all follow downstream. My experience is that a reasonable dose is 25-50 milligrams – I say that because follow-up adrenal stress test results seem to normalise with this dose; however, I may be wrong. Watch this space.

Comprehensive digestive stool analysis (CDSA)

Comprehensive digestive stool analysis looks at the person's ability to digest and absorb together with his/her gut microbes. This is done on a stool sample and can be accessed through my website.

Again, I would not consider using this test until the one-carb meal a day, low GI diet has been well established, together with taking vitamin C to bowel tolerance, and all the above tests are normal.

Details of how to treat the upper fermenting gut can be found in my book *Sustainable Medicine*.[67]

Measures of toxic stress

There is no perfect test which covers all forms of toxic stress – a high index of suspicion is needed. First, have a look at Causes of insulin resistance (page 165) – prescription drugs are common causes of such. Again, establish the low GI diet and do all the above tests first before looking at toxic stress.

a) Toxic elements screen urine following DMSA – This test

can be done on a urine sample. It looks for toxic metals. These are poorly excreted in urine and so to 'see' them, a chelating agent is required. (A chelating agent is one that bonds with metal ions and carries them away with it.) I use DMSA at the rate of 15 milligrams per kilogram body weight. DMSA can be purchased online as 'Captomer' – it is remarkably safe stuff. To do the test, empty the bladder, take the DMSA and collect all urine over the next six hours. Measure the total volume and collect a 10 millilitre sample.

b) Pesticides and volatile organic compounds (VOCs) – I am so fortunate to have access to Acumen tests which I consider to be the most reliable. However, this lab has been overwhelmed by requests so at times we have to look elsewhere. Great Plains Laboratory is offering a test on urine samples for pesticides and VOCs. I do not yet know how reliable this test is, but a fantastic range of pollutants (organophosphates, organochlorines, pyrethroids, phthalates, solvents) is measured and this could be very helpful clinically.

Please note that hair analysis can be misleading. There are often false negative results by which I mean the hair incorrectly shows low levels of toxic mineral when other tests indicate the toxic load is high.

Appendix 10
Doctors are dangerous

After heart disease and cancer, the third most common cause of death is doctors. Dr Barbara Starfield of the Johns Hopkins School of Hygiene and Public Health details how the US health care system may contribute to poor health as follows.[68]

Deaths per year in the USA due to:

- unnecessary surgery – 12,000
- medication errors in hospitals – 7000
- other errors in hospitals – 20,000
- infections in hospitals – 80,000
- non-error, negative effects of drugs – 106,000.

These figures total 225,000 deaths per year from iatrogenic (doctor caused) problems. (Please see Wikipedia for more on Dr Starfield – a remarkable woman.)

To this list I would add problems arising from malnutrition in hospitals, radiation from medical investigations (mammography is a particular concern), unnecessary cancer treatments and the many unrecognised complications of vaccinations. In addition, doctors have the potential to worsen heart disease and cancer through relying on symptom-suppressing medication to manage the symptoms of these diseases instead of addressing the underlying causes. Often this results in late diagnosis – so much so that in the UK, GPs (family doctors) have been offered financial inducements to diagnose dementia. Much more on this subject can be found in my book *Sustainable Medicine*.[67]

Appendix 11
Vital statistics

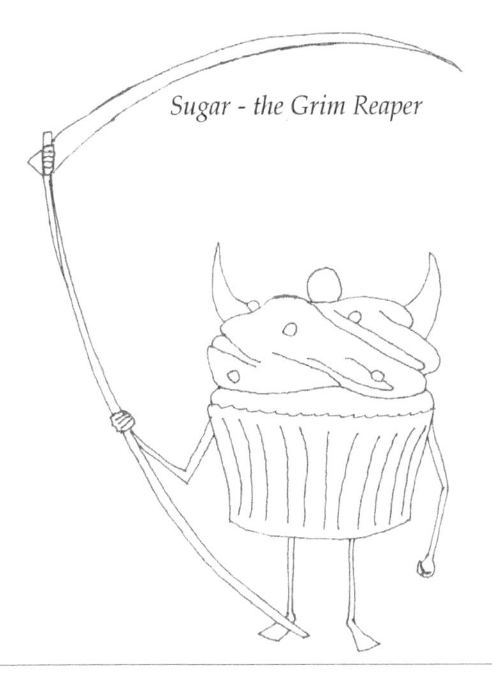

(Vital statistics are not what you think! Craig recalls one of his mathematics masters at Aylesbury Grammar School [an all-boys school, founded in 1598], introducing the topic of inflexions within differential calculus thus – 'The female form has three points of inflexion: the bust, the waist and the hips. Now that I have your attention, let's do the maths!' Here we are talking about other vital statistics…)

Prevalence of diabetes

- More than one million people in the UK were thought to have undiagnosed type 2 diabetes in 2010, double the previous estimate, according to Diabetes Health Intelligence.[69]
- According to Grundy, already in 2008, in most countries between 20% and 30% of the adult population could be characterised as having the metabolic syndrome (the forerunner to diabetes).[70]

Deaths related to diabetes

- Each year in the UK, 24,000 people with diabetes die early – that is, every year, 75,000 people with diabetes die, but of that number, 24,000 die earlier than we would expect for their age group/demographic (HSCIC, 2011).[71]

Cancer and diabetes

- 'Cancer and diabetes are diagnosed within the same individual more frequently than would be expected by chance, even after adjusting for age' (Giovannucci et al, 2010).[72]
- 'Diabetes has been known to increase the risk of cancer for over a century' (Pandey et al, 2011).[73]
- People with type 1 or type 2 diabetes are diagnosed with more of some types of cancer, and are more likely to die from cancer, than people without diabetes. The Australian study which concluded this, included 953,382 registrants from the National Diabetes Service Scheme (NDSS) in Australia: 80,676 with type 1 diabetes and 872,706 with type 2 diabetes, diagnosed between the years 1997 and 2008 (Harding et al, 2014).[74]

Heart disease and stroke in relation to diabetes

- If you have diabetes, you are at least twice as likely as someone who does not have diabetes to have heart disease or a stroke (NIH, 2015).[75]
- People with type 2 diabetes have a two-fold increased risk of stroke within the first five years after diagnosis compared with the general population (Emerging Risk Factors Collaboration (2010) and Jeerakathil et al, 2007).[76,77]

Dementia and diabetes

- People with type 2 diabetes are at a 1.5–2.5-fold increased risk of dementia (Strachan et al, 2011).[78]

Amputations and diabetes

- Over 100 amputations are carried out every week in the UK on people with diabetes because of complications connected with their condition (Holman et al, 2012 and HSCIC, 2013).[79,80]

Blindness and diabetes

- Diabetes is the leading cause of blindness in people of working age in the UK (Kohner et al, 1996 and Arun et al, 2003).[81,82]
- In the US, as many as 25,000 people go blind each year as a result of diabetic retinopathy (Glaucoma Research Foundation, 2011).[83]

Renal disease and diabetes

- Diabetes is the single most common cause of end stage renal disease requiring dialysis or transplant (renal replacement therapies – RRT), with nearly a quarter of all patients having diabetes recorded as the primary cause of their kidney failure and a third of all patients starting RRT having diabetes. For those undergoing RRT, survival rates for patients with diabetes are lower than for people without the condition (3.4 years versus 6.5 years).

- People with diabetes are nearly three times as likely to need RRT as the general population (Gilg et al, 2012; Shaw et al, 2011; Shaw et al, 2012).[84, 85, 86]

Chronic pain and diabetes

- Chronic painful neuropathy (nerve damage) is estimated to affect up to 26% of people with diabetes (Ziegler, 2010).[87]

Hospital admission complications

- In relation to hospital admission, there is a 75.7% increased risk of angina, a 55.1% increased risk of myocardial infarction (heart attack), a 73.2% increased risk of heart failure and a 34.1% increased risk of stroke among people with diabetes (HSCIC, 2011).[88]

Long-term disability and diabetes

- One in every four care home residents has diabetes (Diabetes UK, 2010).[89]

The financial cost of diabetes

- In the UK diabetes costs the NHS £10 billion each year, at the time of writing.
- Diabetes accounts for about 10 % of the NHS budget and 80 % of these costs are due to complications.

Appendix 12
Ketogenic diet for the severely disabled and those with no time to cook

The ketogenic diet can be followed without any cooking and even if the individual is suffering severe disability. The idea behind this Appendix is to provide a list of meal and food suggestions that require no preparation or cooking. In essence, this can be a temporary measure until you can cook more independently/have more time, so don't think that this will have to be your diet forever.

In this Appendix we have included a generalised shopping list, seven days' worth of meal suggestions, and finally a weekly shopping list. The weekly shopping list covers all the foods needed for the seven days of ketogenic meal suggestions that precede it.

GENERALISED SHOPPING LIST (no cooking or food preparation required)

Initially do not worry too much about the protein content – some people can get into ketosis with a high-protein diet. If you can't, then you may need to think about reducing your intake of protein.

Note that in the list that follows, the dietary data are most usually taken from the USDA (United States Department of Agriculture) Database Entry, or otherwise, where there is a proprietary brand, from that brand's nutritional label.

Food	kCal per 100 grams	Carbo-hydrates (grams) per 100 grams (NB: excludes fibre)	Fat (grams) per 100 grams	Fibre (grams) per 100 grams	Protein (grams) per 100 grams
Tinned ham	112	1.1	7.1	0.1	11.0
Tinned gammon	100	1.3	2.5	Trace	18.0
Corned beef	225	1.1	13.5	0.1	24.8
Chopped pork	207	0.6	15.5	0.1	16.9
Tinned sardines in olive oil – boneless	225	0.0	15.4	0.1	21.7
Tinned sardines in tomato juice	142	1.5	7.5	Trace	17.0
Grilled sardines in a tin	198	0.0	11.9	Trace	22.8
Tinned tuna chunks in spring water	113	0.0	0.5	Trace	27.0
Tinned tuna chunks in brine	113	0.0	0.5	Trace	27.0
Tinned tuna chunks in olive oil	209	0.0	9.2	0.0	18.4
Tinned yellow-fin tuna in olive oil	180	Trace	8.0	Trace	27.0
Tinned mackerel in tomato and basil sauce	132	5.7	6.3	Trace	12.8

Food	kCal per 100 grams	Carbo-hydrates (grams) per 100 grams (NB: excludes fibre)	Fat (grams) per 100 grams	Fibre (grams) per 100 grams	Protein (grams) per 100 grams
Tinned steam-cooked mackerel in olive oil	260	0.0	20.0	Trace	20.0
Tinned grilled mackerel fillet	245	0.0	17.0	Trace	23.0
Tinned pink salmon in water	131	Trace	5.4	Trace	20.4
Tinned red salmon in water	151	Trace	7.8	Trace	20.4
Tinned pilchards in tomato sauce	159	2.4	10.1	Trace	14.5
Cornish pilchard fillets in olive oil	205	0.5	13.0	Trace	22.0
Cornish pilchard fillets in tomato sauce	161	1.8	9.1	Trace	18.0
Milano salami	347	0.5	27.3	0.0	24.8
German pepper salami	319	0.7	25.3	1.1	21.5
Serious pig snacking salami	422	0.0	32.7	0.0	32.0
Coyo natural coconut yoghurt	182	0.5	19.0	Trace	3.0

Food	kCal per 100 grams	Carbo-hydrates (grams) per 100 grams (NB: excludes fibre)	Fat (grams) per 100 grams	Fibre (grams) per 100 grams	Protein (grams) per 100 grams
Coyo vanilla coconut yoghurt	182	0.5	19.0	Trace	3.0
Coyo chocolate coconut yoghurt	196	3.9	19.0	Trace	2.3
Coyo cherry coconut yoghurt	177	5.9	16.0	Trace	2.6
Coyo mango coconut yoghurt	177	5.7	16.0	Trace	2.6
Biona organic creamed coconut	664	24.0	68.0	14.0	6.0
Alpro soya yoghurt – plain	50	2.1	2.3	1.0	4.0
Alpro pineapple peach and passionfruit soya yoghurt	78	10.3	1.9	0.8	3.6
Alpro strawberry and rhubarb soya yoghurt	74	9.4	1.9	1.0	3.6
Alpro vanilla yoghurt	75	9.5	2.2	1.0	3.7

Food	kCal per 100 grams	Carbo-hydrates (grams) per 100 grams (NB: excludes fibre)	Fat (grams) per 100 grams	Fibre (grams) per 100 grams	Protein (grams) per 100 grams
Pistachios – roasted and salted	562	18.0	45.0	10.0	20.0
Almonds	576	10.0	49.0	12.0	21.0
Roasted salted peanuts	567	7.0	49.0	9.0	26.0
Salted cashews	553	26.7	44.0	3.3	18.0
Brazil nuts	656	4.0	66.0	8.0	14.0
Hazelnut kernels	628	7.0	61.0	10.0	15.0
Pecans	690	4.0	72.0	10.0	9.0
Pine nuts	673	9.3	68.0	3.7	14.0
Walnuts	654	7.0	65.0	7.0	15.0
Chia seeds	486	8.0	31.0	34.0	17.0
Organic hemp seeds	455	2.8	31.8	30.6	24.0
Pomegranate seeds	100	18.7	1.2	4.0	1.7
Organic flax seed	534	2.0	42.0	27.0	18.0
Pumpkin seeds	446	36.0	19.0	18.0	19.0
Sunflower seeds	584	11.0	51.0	9.0	21.0
Sesame seeds	573	11.0	50.0	12.0	18.0
Macadamia nut butter	711	13.7	65.0	9.0	7.8

Food	kCal per 100 grams	Carbo-hydrates (grams) per 100 grams (NB: excludes fibre)	Fat (grams) per 100 grams	Fibre (grams) per 100 grams	Protein (grams) per 100 grams
Almond butter	640	19.8	50.2	10.1	18.0
Hazelnut butter	693	16.2	60.1	9.1	13.0
Cashew butter	628	18.9	51.3	4.3	20.6
Peanut butter	599	16.8	46.2	6.7	25.6
Coconut butter	670	7.3	64.5	16.3	6.9
90% Lindt dark chocolate	594	16.5	52.8	13.2	10.0
99% Lindt dark chocolate	540	8.0	50.0	6.0	14.0
Green and Black's 85% dark chocolate	630	22.5	53.5	11.5	9.4
Pralus – Le 100% dark chocolate	610	18.0	56.0	13.0	9.0
Avocado	160	2.0	15.0	7.0	2.0
Mayonnaise	680	0.6	75.0	0.0	1.0
Salad cream	336	24.0	27.0	0.3	1.6
Sauerkraut	19	1.4	0.0	2.8	0.7
Tomatoes	18	2.7	0.2	1.2	0.9
Lettuce	15	1.6	0.2	1.3	1.4
Cucumber	16	3.1	0.1	0.3	0.7

SEVEN-DAY MEAL PLAN

Day 1: Ketogenic meal suggestions

Please note, when following the plan below, that for breakfasts, where there is advice to mix seeds with coyo or Alpro yoghurt, different people will have different tastes as to how 'thick' they would like this to be. Please adjust the amount of seeds you mix in to your own taste, but do make sure that you eat all the seeds.

BREAKFAST: DAY 1

Food	Protein (grams)	Carbohydate (grams)	Calories (kCal)
Coyo natural yoghurt (125 grams)	4.0	0.6	228
Mix in 100 grams of chia seeds	17.0	8.0	486
1 slice of linseed bread (see Recipes, page 136) (Approx. amounts)	5.0	0.5	125
With some macadamia nut butter spread on this slice (say, 10 grams)	2.0	1.35	70
Total	28.0	10.45	909

LUNCH: DAY 1

Food	Protein (grams)	Carbohydate (grams)	Calories (kCal)
Tinned mackerel in basil and tomato sauce (120 grams)	15.36	6.84	158
Two avocados (say, 200 grams)	4.0	4.0	320
Frozen berries from the freezer – 50 grams of blueberries	0.3	6.7	30
Total	19.66	17.54	508

MID-AFTERNOON SNACK: DAY 1 (But try to avoid snacking)

Food	Protein (grams)	Carbohydate (grams)	Calories (kCal)
Salami – Serious Pig snacking (50 grams) (see page 132)	16.0	0.0	211
Total	16.0	0.0	211

SUPPER: DAY 1

Food	Protein (grams)	Carbohydate (grams)	Calories (kCal)
Tinned tuna in spring water (120 grams)	32.4	Trace	135
50 grams each of tomato,	0.45	1.35	9
cucumber,	0.7	0.8	8
lettuce	0.35	1.65	8
Dollop mayonnaise (10 grams) (see Recipes, page 137)	0.1	Trace	68
Pine nuts (20 grams)	2.8	1.9	135
Total	36.8	5.7	363

DRINKS

Sparkling water as necessary; maximum of three cups of tea/coffee. (All negligible for carbs.)

TOTALS FOR DAY 1:

Calories – 1991 kCal

Carbs – 33.69 grams

Protein – 100.46 grams

Day 2: Ketogenic meal suggestions

BREAKFAST: DAY 2

Food	Protein (grams)	Carbohydate (grams)	Calories (kCal)
Alpro vanilla yoghurt (200 grams)	7.4	19.0	150
Mix in 100 grams of hemp seeds	24.0	2.8	455
1 slice of linseed bread (see Recipes, page 136) (Approx. amounts)	5.0	0.5	125
With some hazelnut nut butter spread on this slice (say, 10 grams)	1.3	1.6	63
Total	37.7	23.9	793

LUNCH: DAY 2

Food	Protein (grams)	Carbohydate (grams)	Calories (kCal)
Chopped pork (200 gram tin)	33.8	1.2	414
50 grams each of tomato,	0.45	1.35	9
cucumber,	0.7	0.8	8
lettuce	0.35	1.65	8
Frozen berries from freezer – 50 grams of strawberries	0.35	3.0	17
Total	35.65	8.0	456

MID-AFTERNOON SNACK: DAY 2 (But try to avoid snacking)

Food	Protein (grams)	Carbohydate (grams)	Calories (kCal)
One half bar Green and Black's 85% chocolate	4.7	11.25	315
Total	4.7	11.25	315

SUPPER: DAY 2

Food	Protein (grams)	Carbohydate (grams)	Calories (kCal)
Tinned grilled sardines (120 grams)	27.36	0.0	237
One avocado (say 100 grams)	2.0	2.0	160
Total	29.36	2.0	397

DRINKS

Sparkling water as necessary; maximum of three cups of tea/coffee. (All negligible for carbs.)

TOTALS FOR DAY 2:

Calories – 1961 kCal

Carbs – 45.15 grams

Protein – 107.41 grams

Day 3: Ketogenic meal suggestions

BREAKFAST: DAY 3

Food	Protein (grams)	Carbohydate (grams)	Calories (kCal)
Coyo chocolate coconut yoghurt (125 grams)	2.9	4.9	245
Mix in 50 grams of pumpkin seeds	9.5	18.0	223
1 slice of linseed bread (see Recipes, page 134) (Approx. amounts)	5.0	0.5	125
With some peanut nut butter spread on this slice (say, 10 grams)	2.6	1.7	60

Pine nuts (20 grams)	2.8	1.9	135
Total	22.8	27.0	788

LUNCH: DAY 3

Food	Protein (grams)	Carbohydate (grams)	Calories (kCal)
Tinned gammon (200 grams)	36.0	2.6	200
Sauerkraut (pot 100 grams)	0.7	1.4	19
Alpro soya yoghurt, plain (150 grams)	6.0	3.15	75
Almonds (30 grams)	6.3	3.0	172
Total	49.0	10.15	466

MID-AFTERNOON SNACK DAY 3 (But try to avoid snacking)

Food	Protein (grams)	Carbohydate (grams)	Calories (kCal)
Pecans (50 grams)	4.5	2.0	345
Total	4.5	2.0	345

SUPPER: DAY 3

Food	Protein (grams)	Carbohydate (grams)	Calories (kCal)
Corned beef (125 gram tin)	31.0	1.38	282
50 grams each of tomato,	0.45	1.35	9
cucumber,	0.7	0.8	8
lettuce	0.35	1.65	8
Dollop mayonnaise (10 grams) (see Recipes, page 137)	0.1	Trace	68
Total	32.6	5.18	375

DRINKS

Sparkling water as necessary; maximum of three cups of tea/ coffee. (All negligible for carbs.)

TOTALS FOR DAY 3:

Calories –1974 kCal

Carbs – 44.33 grams

Protein – 108.9 grams

Day 4: Ketogenic meal suggestions

BREAKFAST: DAY 4

Food	Protein (grams)	Carbohydate (grams)	Calories (kCal)
Alpro strawberry and rhubarb yoghurt (150 grams)	5.4	14.1	111
Mix in 150 grams sunflower seeds	31.5	16.5	876
1 slice of linseed bread (see Recipes, page 136) (Approx. amounts)	5.0	0.5	125
Total	41.9	31.1	1112

LUNCH: DAY 4

Food	Protein (grams)	Carbohydate (grams)	Calories (kCal)
Tinned ham (125 gram tin)	13.75	1.38	140
2 avocados (say 200 grams)	4.0	4.0	320
Frozen berries from freezer – 50 grams of raspberries	0.6	2.5	26
Total	18.35	7.88	486

MID-AFTERNOON SNACK DAY 4 (But try to avoid snacking)

Food	Protein (grams)	Carbohydate (grams)	Calories (kCal)
Serious Pig salami (25 grams) (see page 132)	8.0	0.0	106
Total	8.0	0.0	106

SUPPER: DAY 4

Food	Protein (grams)	Carbohydate (grams)	Calories (kCal)
Tinned sardines in tomato juice (125 gram tin)	21.25	1.9	178
50 grams each of tomato,	0.45	1.35	9
cucumber,	0.7	0.8	8
lettuce	0.35	1.65	8
Dollop mayonnaise (say, 20 grams) (see Recipes, page 137)	0.3	4.8	67
Total	23.05	10.5	270

DRINKS

Sparkling water as necessary; maximum of three cups of tea/coffee. (All negligible for carbs.)

TOTALS FOR DAY 4:

Calories – 1974 kCal

Carbs – 49.48 grams

Protein – 91.3 grams

Day 5: Ketogenic meal suggestions

BREAKFAST: DAY 5

Food	Protein (grams)	Carbohydate (grams)	Calories (kCal)
Coyo, pineapple, peach and passionfruit yoghurt (125 gram pot)	4.5	12.9	97
Mix in 100 grams sesame seeds	18.0	11.0	573
1 slice of linseed bread (see Recipes, page 136) (Approx. amounts)	5.0	0.5	125
With some cashew butter spread on this slice (say, 10 grams)	2.1	1.9	63
Total	29.6	26.3	858

LUNCH: DAY 5

Food	Protein (grams)	Carbohydate (grams)	Calories (kCal)
Tinned red salmon (150 grams)	30.6	Trace	227
50 grams each of tomato,	0.45	1.35	9
cucumber,	0.7	0.8	8
lettuce	0.35	1.65	8
Dollop mayonnaise (20 grams) (see Recipes, page 137)	0.2	Trace	136
Hazelnuts (10 grams)	1.5	0.7	63
Total	33.8	4.5	451

MID-AFTERNOON SNACK: DAY 5 (But try to avoid snacking)

Food	Protein (grams)	Carbohydate (grams)	Calories (kCal)
90% Lindt dark chocolate (50 grams)	5.0	8.25	297
Total	5.0	8.25	297

SUPPER: DAY 5

Food	Protein (grams)	Carbohydate (grams)	Calories (kCal)
Milano salami (75 grams)	18.6	0.38	260
Sauerkraut (200 grams)	1.4	2.8	38
Total	20.0	3.18	298

DRINKS

Sparkling water as necessary; maximum of three cups of tea/coffee. (All negligible for carbs.)

TOTALS FOR DAY 5:

Calories – 1904 kCal
Carbs – 42.23 grams
Protein – 88.4 grams

Day 6: Ketogenic meal suggestions

BREAKFAST: DAY 6

Food	Protein (grams)	Carbohydate (grams)	Calories (kCal)
Alpro vanilla yoghurt (150 grams)	5.55	14.25	112
Mix in 100 grams flax seed	18.0	2.0	534
1 slice of linseed bread (see Recipes, page 136) (Approx. amounts)	5.0	0.5	125

With some coconut butter spread on this slice (say, 10 grams)	0.7	0.7	67
Total	29.25	17.45	838

LUNCH: DAY 6

Food	Protein (grams)	Carbohydate (grams)	Calories (kCal)
Corned beef (125 gram tin)	31.0	1.38	282
50 grams each of tomato,	0.45	1.35	9
cucumber,	0.7	0.8	8
lettuce	0.35	1.65	8
Dollop mayonnaise (say, 10 grams) (see Recipes, page 137)	0.1	Trace	68
Pine nuts (20 grams)	2.8	1.9	135
Total	35.4	7.08	510

MID-AFTERNOON SNACK DAY 6 (But try to avoid snacking)

Food	Protein (grams)	Carbohydate (grams)	Calories (kCal)
Brazil nuts (40 grams)	5.6	1.6	262
Total	5.6	1.6	262

SUPPER: DAY 6

Food	Protein (grams)	Carbohydate (grams)	Calories (kCal)
Cornish pilchards in tomato sauce (120 gram tin)	17.4	2.88	190
One avocado (say, 100 grams)	2.0	2.0	160

Sauerkraut (200 grams)	1.4	2.8	38
Total	20.8	7.68	388

DRINKS

Sparkling water as necessary; maximum of three cups of tea/coffee. (All negligible for carbs.)

TOTALS FOR DAY 6:

Calories – 1998 kCal

Carbs – 33.81 grams

Protein – 91.05 grams

Day 7: Ketogenic meal suggestions

BREAKFAST: DAY 7

Food	Protein (grams)	Carbohydate (grams)	Calories (kCal)
Alpro soya yoghurt, plain (150 grams)	6.0	3.15	75
Mix with 100 grams chia seeds	17.0	8.0	486
1 slice of linseed bread (see Recipes, page 134) (Approx. amounts)	5.0	0.5	125
With some macadamia nut butter spread on this slice (say, 10 gram)	2.0	1.35	70
Pine nuts (20 grams)	2.8	1.9	135
Total	32.8	14.9	891

LUNCH: DAY 7

Food	Protein (grams)	Carbohydate (grams)	Calories (kCal)
Chopped pork (200 gram tin)	33.8	1.2	414
50 grams each of tomato,	0.45	1.35	9
cucumber,	0.7	0.8	8
lettuce	0.35	1.65	8
Frozen berries from freezer – 50 grams of gooseberries	0.45	2.85	22
Total	35.75	7.85	461

MID-AFTERNOON SNACK DAY 7 (But try to avoid snacking)

Food	Protein (grams)	Carbohydate (grams)	Calories (kCal)
Walnuts (50 grams)	7.5	3.5	327
Total	7.5	3.5	327

SUPPER: DAY 7

Food	Protein (grams)	Carbohydate (grams)	Calories (kCal)
Tinned tuna in spring water (120 grams)	32.4	Trace	135
50 grams each of tomato,	0.45	1.35	9
cucumber,	0.7	0.8	8
lettuce	0.35	1.65	8
Dollop mayonnaise (say, 10 grams) (see Recipes, page 137)	0.1	Trace	68
Sauerkraut (200 grams)	1.4	2.8	38
Total	35.4	6.60	266

DRINKS

Sparkling water as necessary; maximum of three cups of tea/coffee. (All negligible for carbs.)

TOTALS FOR DAY 7:

Calories – 1945 kCal
Carbs – 32.85 grams
Protein – 111.45 grams

Weekly shopping list for meal suggestions Days 1 to 7

(One loaf of linseed bread as on page 136. Use 250 grams of linseed and scale the other ingredients up. This is the only item that needs cooking.)

Coyo natural yoghurt (125 grams)
Coyo chocolate coconut yoghurt (125 grams)
Coyo pineapple, peach and passionfruit yoghurt (125 grams)
Alpro vanilla yoghurt (200 grams) and Alpro vanilla yoghurt (150 grams)
2 x Alpro soya yoghurt, plain (150 grams)
Alpro strawberry and rhubarb yoghurt (150 grams)

Tinned mackerel in basil and tomato sauce (120 grams)
Tinned tuna in spring water (120 grams)
Tinned grilled sardines (120 grams)
Tinned tuna in spring water (120 grams)
Tinned red salmon (150 grams)
Tinned Cornish pilchards in tomato sauce (120 grams)
Tinned sardines in tomato juice (125 grams)
2 x tins chopped pork (200 gram tins)
Tinned gammon (200 grams)

2 x tins corned beef (125 gram tins)
Tinned ham (125 grams)
Salami – Serious Pig Snacking (100 grams) (see page 132)
Milano salami (75 grams)
6 avocados
400 grams each of tomato, cucumber, lettuce
Sauerkraut (700 grams)

100 grams of flax seeds
100 grams of sesame seeds
150 grams of sunflower seeds
100 grams of hemp seeds
100 grams of chia seeds
50 grams of pumpkin seeds
60 grams of pine nuts
30 grams of almonds
50 grams of pecans
10 grams of hazelnuts
40 grams of Brazil nuts
50 grams of walnuts

50 grams of blueberries
50 grams of strawberries
50 grams of raspberries
50 grams of gooseberries

1 bar Green and Black's 85% chocolate – will last two weeks
1 bar 90% Lindt dark chocolate – will last two weeks

Pot mayonnaise – will last more than one week
Pot salad cream – will last more than one week
Pot macadamia nut butter – will last more than one week
Pot hazelnut nut butter – will last more than one week
Pot peanut nut butter spread – will last more than one week

Pot cashew butter spread – will last more than one week
Pot coconut butter – will last more than one week

CONCLUSION

These are meal suggestions only and demonstrate how you can construct 'low effort' ketogenic diets from the information and tables in Chapter 7, Prevention, treatment and reversal of metabolic syndrome and diabetes, and from the table above. By way of notes to these meal suggestions:

- Please feel free to add 'taste enhancers' from the tables in Chapter 7 (see page 113) so as to add variety.
- These meal suggestions require one loaf of linseed bread (recipe as described in Appendix 1, page 136) to be cooked once a week. It is hoped that this task can be done by a carer or friend.
- Obviously, one can mix up a breakfast from one day with a lunch from another and so on, as long as one sticks to the overall guidelines.
- In these meals, the 50 grams of carbs and 2000 kCal of calories limits have been adhered to. The protein levels have been kept to around 100 grams. This is less than noted in Chapter 7 and so you could divert some of your dietary intake into more protein-rich foods. Protein can be converted into carbs and so having low amounts of protein is protective against this.
- A small afternoon snack has been included on each day. This is because it is recognised that initially it will be difficult to avoid such snacking 'habits'. This is not ideal, and so, as time goes by, try to drop the snack and add in equivalent amounts of protein, carbs and calories to the main meals.
- Those who are concerned about soy products should stick to the Coyo breakfast option for the time being until they

are able to move forward with cooking.

- There is an alternative to the Alpro yoghurt – Provamel, which is sugar free and so some individuals may prefer this in their individual circumstances.
- If you feel that 2000 kCal is too high for your personal level of activity then cutting out the snacks each day will help to reduce the calorific intake.

Postscript

Western Medicine has lost its way. Doctors no longer look for the underlying causes of disease, a process which used to be called diagnosis, but rather seek a 'quick fix' response that will see the patient out of their surgery door in under 10 minutes. This quick-fix response usually comprises the prescribing of symptom-suppressing medications. Doctors have become the puppets of Big Pharma, dishing out drugs and working to a 'checklist' culture which is directed at the symptom, rather than the patient. Patients are seen as a collection of walking symptoms, rather than as people, each with a highly individual set of circumstances. Worse than this, not only do these prescription drugs do nothing to address the root causes of illness, but often they accelerate the underlying pathology as well as having unwanted side effects, and so drug prescribing snowballs. This leads to a vicious spiral of increasing drug costs coupled with worsening pathologies for individual patients, whilst at the same time the number of new, and chronic, patients increases because the root causes of their illnesses are never properly addressed. It is no wonder that the National Health Service is being overwhelmed. The result is that millions suffer a painful, premature, and often lingering, death from diseases which are completely avoidable and reversible.

The time has come for patients to be empowered to take back control of their own health. To achieve this empowerment, patients need:

1. The knowledge to work out why they have symptoms and disease.
2. Direct access to all relevant medical tests.
3. Direct access to knowledgeable therapists who can further advise and guide them, together with direct access to safe and effective remedies.

None of this is beyond patients who are always highly motivated to be well again, and who of course know their bodies better than anyone else. It is time to break down the artificial barriers that have been placed between patients and the medical knowledge, tests and experts that they so deserve.

This three-stage process of patient emancipation can be achieved by following the steps below.

1. The knowledge can be found in these three books:

a) *Sustainable Medicine* – This is the starting point for treating all symptoms and diseases. It explains why we have symptoms, such as fatigue and pain, and details how one can work out the mechanisms of such symptoms. It also explains which are the appropriate medical tests to diagnose these mechanisms. Most importantly, *Sustainable Medicine* identifies the 'tools of the trade' to effect a cure. These tools include diets, nutritional supplements and natural remedies.

b) *Diabetes – delicious diets, not dangerous drugs* – All medical therapies should start with diet. Modern Western diets are driving our modern epidemics of diabetes, heart disease, cancer and dementia; this process is called metabolic syndrome. *Diabetes* explains in detail why and how we have arrived at a situation where the *real* weapons of mass destruction can be found in our kitchens. Importantly, it describes the vital steps every one of us can make to reverse the situation so that life can be lived to its full potential.

c) *Chronic Fatigue Syndrome – it's mitochondria not hypochondria* – This book further explores the commonest symptom which people complain of – namely, fatigue – together with its pathological end result when this symptom is ignored. This is my life's work, having spent over 35 years in clinical practice plus many months in academic research and co-authored three scientific papers, all directed at solving this jigsaw of an illness. This book has application not just for the severely fatigued patient but also for the athlete looking for peak performance.

2. Access to medical tests

As I have said earlier, patients need to be given control of their own medical tests. Many relevant tests can be accessed directly through:

- Academy of Nutritional Medicine at www.aonm.org/Armin%20Labs
- Bio Lab at www.biolab.co.uk (needs a referral from a health practitioner – see NHS below)
- Genova labs at www.gdx.net/uk (for stool, urine and saliva testing – needs a referral from a health practitioner – see NHS below)
- The Doctors' Laboratory at www.tdlpathology.com (needs a referral from a doctor – see NHS below)

Tests available include blood, urine, stool and saliva samples. Many blood tests can be carried out at home on a finger-drop sample of blood, without the need for a nurse or doctor to be involved at all.

3. Direct access to knowledgeable therapists who can further advise and guide patients

The Natural Health Service International (www.thenhsi.com) is a website where any knowledgeable healthcare practitioner (medical doctor, alternative therapist or expert patient) can offer his/her opinion to any patient. This opinion may be free, or for a consultation fee, and may be made by telephone, email, Skype or a face-to-face consultation. The practitioner needs no premises or support staff since bookings and payments are made online. Patients give feedback to that practitioner's reputation page and star ratings evolve.

Glossary

Acid-alkali balance

Maintaining the correct acidity / alkalinity (or pH) of the blood is an essential part of good health. Acidity / alkalinity is determined by the concentration of hydrogen ions – that is, the lower the pH, the greater the acidity and the greater the concentration of hydrogen ions. It is important to realise the pH scale is a logarithmic one. This means that the difference between a pH of 7 and 4 means a thousand-fold increase in hydrogen ions. (For the mathematically minded, this is calculated, in this case, as 7-4 = 3 and then raising 10 to the power of 3, giving 1000.) Such a shift would have a massive effect on biochemical processes, most of which are exquisitely sensitive to pH changes. For normal metabolism, the pH of the blood is tightly controlled by the lungs and the kidneys. In the short term, the lungs compensate where there is a tendency to acidosis (increased acidity) by slowing breathing and thereby retaining carbon dioxide and increasing bicarbonate, and with that, the pH. In the medium term, the kidneys compensate – where there is acidosis, we pee out acid.

This works fine when we have enough acid or bicarbonate to play with. We run into problems when we don't. Where there is poor mitochondrial function, we slip into anaerobic metabolism and produce lactic acid. This chronic overproduction puts us into a permanently acidic state, which means that any person with a tendency to fatigue and anaerobic metabolism is likely to be chronically acidotic. We try to correct this by peeing out acid, but there is only so much we can do.

I suspect the upper fermenting gut results in an acidosis – sugars may be fermented into acids, such as D-lactate, to cause D-lactate acidosis.

The possible effects of being acidic are:

- Hypoglycaemia – An acidic body means we cannot release glucose from the liver, nor can we make use of sugar in blood and muscle (glycolysis, that is the conversion of glucose, is inhibited). So mitochondria are further starved of energy and the sufferer craves carbs, feeling ghastly when s/he does not eat.
- Muscles contract less strongly
- Acid urine strips out minerals so we lose minerals too easily. Acidic urine is a risk factor for osteoporosis.
- Plasma potassium levels may rise.

Hyperventilation will worsen any tendency to acidosis because it washes out carbon dioxide, and therefore bicarbonate, from the blood.

http://www.drmyhill.co.uk/wiki/Acid-Alkali_balance

Acquired metabolic dyslexias

As we age, just like an ageing car, we become less efficient in three respects. Firstly, we need more raw materials as our ability to digest and absorb declines. Those that I currently believe need to be supplemented in supra-physiological doses include vitamin B12 1 milligram (mg), vitamin B3 500 mg, vitamin D 2000 iu and vitamin C 2 grams. There may well be others. Secondly, our ability to synthesise key molecules from raw materials declines. My list of such so far includes melatonin (the sleep hormone – 3 mg), adrenal hormones (such as pregnenolone [50 mg], possibly, and DHEA), co-enzyme Q-10 (200 mg) and D-ribose (5 grams).

Again, there may well be others as I learn more. Thirdly, we need additional help with detoxification since we live in an increasingly toxic world. I consider glutathione (250 mg daily) to be essential.

Adrenal gland problems

The adrenal glands are the 'gear box' of our car responsible for matching energy demand with energy consumption. They are additionally responsible for controlling the amount of inflammation in the body. They achieve this by secreting adrenaline (the short-term response, measured in seconds and minutes), followed by cortisol (a medium-term response measured in minutes and hours), followed by DHEA (dehydroepiandrosterone – a longer-term stress hormone).

The Hungarian physiologist Hans Selye showed that if you stressed rats, their adrenal glands enlarged to produce more stress hormones (including cortisol and DHEA) to allow the rat to cope with that stress. If the rat had a break and a rest, then the adrenal gland would return to its normal size and recover. However, if the rat was stressed without a break or a rest, he would be apparently all right for some time, but then suddenly collapsed and died. When Selye looked at the adrenal glands at this point, they were shrivelled up. The glands had become exhausted.

The current Western way of life is for people to push themselves more and more. Many can cope with a great deal of stress, but everybody has their breaking point. The adrenal glands are responsible for the body's hormonal response to this stress. They produce adrenaline, which stimulates the instant stress hormone response ('fight or flight' reaction), and cortisol and DHEA, which create the short- and long-term stress hormone responses respectively. When the glands become exhausted, chronic fatigue develops and tests of adrenal function typically show low levels of cortisol and DHEA. DHEA has only recently been studied because it had not been realised that it had any important actions.

All steroid hormone synthesis starts with cholesterol. The first biochemical step takes place in mitochondria where there is a conversion to pregnenolone. The body can then shunt from pregnenolone into either a stress or catabolic mode (to cortisol) or a rebuilding mode (anabolic hormones such as DHEA, testosterone and oestrogen).

Both anabolism (building up tissues) and catabolism (breaking tissues down) are essential for life in the right amounts: too little causes problems, as does too much. Research suggests this balance protects against the development of osteoporosis, which is a major consideration for anyone unable to exercise, including all CFS sufferers.

http://drmyhill.co.uk/wiki/Common_Hormonal_Problems_in_CFS_-_Adrenal

Adrenaline (epinephrine)

Adrenaline is the instant stress response hormone that drives our fight or flight reaction. This reaction is characterised by intense arousal (sometimes to the point of anxiety or panic), with a faster heart rate, high blood pressure, higher blood sugar level and sometimes even minor tremor. This is the stress hormone which allows us to move up a gear, sometimes perhaps into overdrive, even in order to kill, within a stressful situation. An obvious evolutionary cause of such stress would be to be hunted by a predator. In our modern, safer lives, I suspect that the commonest stress is falling blood sugar levels and this release of adrenaline is a central part of metabolic syndrome.

Advanced glycation end products

Sugar is sticky stuff. It sticks onto almost anything, including proteins and fats, and in doing so it de-natures them (that is, permanently changes their physical shape). These de-natured molecules are called AGEs (advanced glycation end products).

Because we all need some sugar in our bloodstream this is an inevitable part of the ageing process. However, it is accelerated if blood sugar levels run high. One example of an AGE is glycated haemoglobin – this is a measure of glucose stuck on to haemoglobin and, therefore, gives us an idea of average blood sugar readings over the last three months. AGEs in the skin cause brown stains – that is, the freckle often associated with aged skin. They are a major cause of arterial damage. Increasingly there is evidence suggesting they stick to proteins in the nervous system to form prions and so drive neurological diseases like Alzheimer's and Parkinson's disease.

Allergy

Allergy is the great mimic. In some ways the immune system is not very clever. It can react to things in only one way – that is, with inflammation. Inflammation causes redness, swelling, pain, heat and loss of function. When you look at a diseased area, you can see those signs, but it does not tell you what is the cause of those signs. So for example, looking at an area of inflamed skin you may not be able to tell if it has been infected, sun-burnt or frozen, had acid spilled on it, or is responding allergically, or whatever. Again, seeing a person with hay fever you may not be able to distinguish this from a head cold. Hay fever sufferers may get a fever too.

You can be allergic to anything under the sun, including the sun. For practical purposes, allergies are split up into allergies to foods, chemicals (including drugs) and inhalants (pollens and microorganisms bacteria, mites, etc).

People with undiagnosed food allergy often initially present with symptoms due to inflammation in the gut (irritable bowel syndrome) and inflammation in the brain (mood swings, depression or brain fog in adults, or hyperactivity in children). However, the inflammation can occur anywhere in the body, resulting in asthma, rhinitis, eczema, arthritis and muscle pain, cystitis or vaginitis, or a combination of symptoms. If the cause is not identified, the inflammation often becomes more generalised, resulting in chronic fatigue.

http://drmyhill.co.uk/wiki/Allergy_to_Foods,_Inhalants_&_

Antioxidants

What allows us to live and our bodies to function are billions of chemical reactions in the body which occur every second. These are essential for the production of energy, which drives all the processes of life such as nervous function, movement, heart function, digestion and so on. If all these enzyme reactions invariably occurred perfectly, there would be no need for an antioxidant system. However, even our own enzyme systems make mistakes and the process of producing energy in mitochondria is highly active. When mistakes occur, free radicals are produced. Essentially, a free radical is a molecule with an unpaired electron; it is highly reactive and to stabilise its own structure, it will literally stick on to anything. That 'anything' could be a cell membrane, a protein, a fat, a piece of DNA, or whatever. In sticking on to something, it denatures that something so that it has to be replaced. This means having free radicals is extremely damaging to the body and therefore the body has evolved a system to mop up these free radicals before they have a chance to do such damage and this is called our antioxidant system.

There are many substances in the body which act as antioxidants, but the three most important frontline antioxidants are:

- **co-enzyme Q10 (Co-Q10)**: This is the most important antioxidant inside mitochondria and also a vital molecule in oxidative phosphorylation. Co-Q10 deficiency may also cause oxidative phosphorylation to go slow because it is the most important receiver and donor of electrons in oxidative phosphorylation. People with low levels of Co-Q10 have low levels of energy.
- **superoxide dismutase (SODase)** is the most important

superoxide scavenger in muscles (zinc and copper SODase inside cells, manganese SODase inside mitochondria and zinc and copper extracellular SODase outside cells), and
- **glutathione peroxidase**: This enzyme is dependent on selenium and glutathione, a three-amino acid polypeptide, and a vital free radical scavenger in the bloodstream.

These molecules are present in parts of a million and are in the frontline process of absorbing free radicals. When they absorb an electron from a free radical, both the free radical and the antioxidant are effectively neutralised, but the antioxidants re-activate themselves by passing that electron back to second line antioxidants such as vitamins A and beta-carotene, some of the B vitamins, vitamin D, vitamin E, vitamin K and probably many others. These are present in parts per thousand. Again, these are neutralised by accepting an electron, but that is then passed back to the ultimate repository of electrons, namely vitamin C. This is present in higher concentrations.

http://drmyhill.co.uk/wiki/Antioxidants

Apoptosis

Apoptosis is a form of cell death in which a cell is eliminated without releasing harmful substances. Mitochondria control this process. It has a crucial role in the health of the body because it removes old cells, unnecessary cells and unhealthy cells. When apoptosis does not happen as it should, then cells that should 'killed' may persist and become 'immortal'; this can result in the start of cancers.

Autoimmunity

Autoimmunity occurs when the immune system has made a mistake. The immune system has a difficult job to do, because it has to distinguish between molecules which are dangerous to the body and molecules which are safe. Sometimes it gets its wires crossed and starts making antibodies against molecules which are 'safe'. For some people this results in allergies, which is a useless inflammation against 'safe' foreign molecules. For others this results in autoimmunity, which is a useless inflammation against the body's own molecules. These are acquired problems – we know that because they become much more common with age. It is likely we are seeing more autoimmunity because of Western lifestyles, diets and pollution.

Chemicals, especially heavy metals, get stuck onto cells and change their 'appearance' to the immune system and thereby switch on inappropriate reactions.

http://drmyhill.co.uk/wiki/Autoimmune_diseases_-_the_environmental_approach_to_treating

Brain fog

What I mean by brain fog is:

- Poor short-term memory;
- Difficulty learning new things;
- Poor mental stamina and concentration – there may be difficulty reading a book or following a film story or following a line of argument;
- Difficulty finding the right word;
- Thinking one word, but saying another.

What allows the brain to work quickly and efficiently is its energy supply. If this is impaired in any way, then the brain will go slow. Initially, the symptoms would be of foggy brain, but if symptoms progress, we end up with dementia. We all see this in our everyday life, with the effect of alcohol being the best example. Short-term exposure gives us a deliciously foggy brain – we stop caring, we stop worrying, it alleviates anxiety. However, it also removes our drive to do things, our ability to remember; it impairs judgement and our ability to think clearly. Medium-term exposure results in moodswings and anxiety (only alleviated by more alcohol). Longer-term use could result in severe depression and then dementia – examples include Korsakoff's psychosis and Wernike's encephalopathy. (Incidentally, these two examples also illustrate how most drug side-effects result from nutritional deficiencies – look them up on Wikipedia!)

The cellular form of energy, ATP, along with DNA, is an ancient molecule. It multitasks. It also functions as a neurotransmitter – to be precise a co-transmitter. Other neurotransmitters will not work unless they are accompanied by a molecule of ATP. Improve ATP and you improve all aspects of brain function. Improving ATP delivery is the best treatment for low mood and depression.

http://www.drmyhill.co.uk/wiki/Brain_fog_-_poor_memory,_difficulty_thinking_clearly_etc

Candida

See Yeast problems, page 257 and:

http://drmyhill.co.uk/wiki/Yeast_problems_and_candida

Carbohydrate

All vegetable material (grains, pulses, vegetables, salads, fruits, berries, nuts and seeds) contain carbohydrates. These are comprised of:

1. Simple monosaccharides and disaccharides. (They all taste sweet and we call them sugars.)
2. Polysaccharides. (These are starches, such as from grain flours or potato.)
3. Complex polysaccharides (which we call vegetable fibre).

The sugars and starches are easily digested in our gut, readily absorbed and their combined effect on blood sugar is approximately given by the glycaemic index (GI) (see page 75).

Vegetable fibre cannot be digested by human enzymes; it must be fermented by friendly bacteria in the large bowel. It is fermented to form short-chain fatty acids, which are a useful fuel for the body but which do not affect blood sugar levels. This is what makes high-fibre vegetables such desirable foods.

The carbohydrate content of a product is usually given as total (or net) carbohydrate which is comprised of dietary fibre, starches and sugars. The starch content may not be listed but can be inferred, as, for example:

Whole-grain brown rice, cooked, contains per 100 grams
Total carbohydrate 23 grams
Dietary fibre 1.8 grams
Sugar 0.4 grams
Ergo, starch 20.8 grams, being 23 minus 1.8 minus 0.4 grams.

However, for practical purposes, when we talk about 'carbs', we mean sugars and starches, not vegetable fibre.

Chemical poisoning

The diagnosis of chemical poisoning is suspected from a history of exposures resulting in typical clinical syndromes and confirmed by the appropriate medical tests. There is a series of criteria to be fulfilled to make a confident clinical diagnosis of poisoning by chemicals. The criteria are:

1. The subject was fit and well prior to chemical exposures.
2. There is evidence of exposure to the putative chemicals and toxins.
3. The subject initially developed local symptoms which became worse with repeated exposures.
4. With repeated exposures a typical clinical picture emerges characterised by chronic fatigue syndrome, immune disruption (allergies, autoimmunity, susceptibility to infections), accelerated ageing (so the sufferer gets diseases before their time), neuro-degeneration, diabetes and cancer.
5. Similar patterns of disease are seen in other people working under similar conditions.

6. There is similar factual evidence from other subjects who have been poisoned, such as the Gulf War veterans, sheepdip poisoned farmers, aerotoxic pilots.
7. There is laboratory evidence of poisoning and effects of that poisoning.
8. There are no other possible explanations for this pattern of symptoms.
9. There is a response to treatment with clinical improvements as a result of detoxification, nutritional and immune support. http://drmyhill.co.uk/wiki/Chemical_poisoning_-_general_principles_of_diagnosis_and_treatment

Co-enzyme Q10
See anti-oxidants (page 214) and http://drmyhill.co.uk/wiki/Antioxidants

Cortisol
Cortisol is a hormone released by the adrenal glands in response to stress. Essentially, adrenaline is the immediate response, cortisol the medium-term response and DHEA the long-term response. Between these three hormones the body can gear up to stress, maintain that stress response for the required duration, then normality is restored as the levels of these hormones drop back to normal.

Detoxification
As part of normal metabolism, the body produces toxins which have to be eliminated, otherwise they poison the system. Therefore, the body has evolved a mechanism for getting rid of these toxins and the methods that it uses are as follows:

- Antioxidant system – for mopping up free radicals. See Antioxidants.
- The liver – detoxification by oxidation and conjugation (amino-acids, sulphur-compounds, glucuronide,

glutathione, etc) for excretion in urine.

- Fat-soluble toxins can be excreted in the bile. The problem here is that many of these are recycled because they are reabsorbed in the gut.
- Sweating – many toxins and heavy metals can be lost through the skin.
- Dumping chemicals in hair, nails and skin, which is then shed.

This system has worked perfectly well for thousands of years. Problems now arise because of toxins which we are absorbing from the outside world. This is inevitable since we live in equilibrium with the outside world. The problem is that these toxins (such as alcohol) may overwhelm the system for detoxification, or they may be impossible to break down (e.g. silicone and organochlorines), or they may get stuck in fatty organs and cell membranes and so not be accessible to the liver for detoxification (for example, many volatile organic compounds). We all carry these toxins as a result of living in our polluted world.

http://drmyhill.co.uk/wiki/Detoxification_-_an_overview

http://drmyhill.co.uk/wiki/Detoxing_-_Far_Infrared_Sauna_(FIRS)

DMSA

This is the chelating agent 2-3-dimercapto-succinic acid magnesium salt, used for heavy metal detox. It binds with metals in the body and takes them with it when excreted.

http://drmyhill.co.uk/wiki/Heavy_metal_poisoning_-_vital_for_autistic_kids_-_think_of_when_all_else_fails!

Energy expenditure

We all have a pot of energy which is available to us to spend over the day. What prevents us spending too much is the symptom of fatigue. We have to spend that pot of energy just to stay alive in 'house keeping' duties, as well as mentally, physically, emotionally or immunologically. If either the pot of energy is too small (because of poor mitochondrial function, poor fuel supply, poor adrenal function, poor thyroid function and so on) or we spend energy wastefully, we can develop chronic fatigue. Of course, the business of pacing is all about spending mental and physical energy judiciously. Many have experienced how energy sapping it is to expend emotional energy. However, I suspect a greatly overlooked cause of wasting of energy is immunological.

http://www.drmyhill.co.uk/wiki/Energy_Expenditure_in_ME/CFS:_Immune_wastage_of_energy_and_Rituximab

Enzyme-potentiated desensitisation (EPD)

Enzyme-potentiated desensitisation (EPD) is a vaccine which can be used to desensitise patients to foods, inhalants and chemicals. It has some bacterial antigens. The vaccine has been developed and refined by Dr Len McEwen over the past 30 years. It is supplied to the doctor who mixes the appropriate dose in a sterile environment, immediately prior to dosing. EPD works by manipulating the normal immune processes for creating and turning off allergies.

http://drmyhill.co.uk/wiki/Enzyme_Potentiated_Desensitisation_(EPD)_-_how_it_works

Exercise

Humans, along with all other mammals, evolved living physically active lives. This usually meant long hours of sustained activity, but there would be occasions when maximal energy output was needed, for example, to fight an enemy or bring down a prey. It could be argued that most internal metabolism is geared towards physical activity and without this we cannot be fully well.

We need exercise as we need food and water: in just the right amount. Too much risks injury and muscle damage; too little and we degenerate. To maintain optimal fitness, we need steady sustained exercise combined with outbursts of extreme energy. Just as with food, the type of exercise and the amount are critical. After research and practical application, Dr Doug McGuff and John Little produced their book *Body by Science – a research-based programme for strength training, body building and complete fitness in 12 minutes a week*. Thanks to their work, we can now see how to exercise most efficiently. We do not want to do so much that we wear out our body (this is what happens with so many athletes – most runners are carrying injuries), but when we do exercise it must be effective to improve cardiovascular fitness. What is so interesting about Little & McGuff's approach is how well this correlates with what we already know about mitochondria, blood sugar control and fats. This approach makes perfect evolutionary sense. I do not see badgers and foxes trotting round my hill every morning to get fit!

Most of the time wild animals are in hiding or feeding quietly. Once a week there will be a predator-prey interaction – the predator must run for his life to get his breakfast, the prey must run for his life! In doing so, both parties will achieve maximal lactic acid burn. This is all that is required to get fit and stay fit.

http://www.drmyhill.co.uk/wiki/Exercise_-_the_right_sort

Far-infrared sauna (FIRS)

Time-honoured methods of detoxification include saunas, Turkish baths and spa therapies, and I recommend all these treatments to my patients. However, the problem with these treatments is that not only do they warm up the skin and subcutaneous tissues, but the whole body is warmed up. This means that chemicals are mobilised from the fat (which largely speaking lies underneath the skin), and, when they get into the bloodstream, can cause acute poisoning.

Many of my patients are therefore unable to tolerate these sweating therapies. Furthermore, many sick CFS patients cannot tolerate heat because this increases demands on the heart. In severe CFS energy delivery to the heart is impaired so it cannot increase its output to cope with the demands of heat.

This is why I became particularly interested in a new technique described in Dr Sherry Rogers' book *Detoxify or Die* (available from Amazon www.amazon.co.uk). She advocates a technique called 'far infrared saunas'. Far-infrared rays constitute the main energy source that comes from the sun and are responsible for warming our skin when we sit in direct sunshine. The rays penetrate several centimetres through the skin and heat up subcutaneous tissues. With enough sun on the skin, the skin will sweat; chemicals from subcutaneous tissues will be mobilised and pass out through sweat. The sunshine does this without heating up the core temperature (although if you lie in the sun for long enough, then your core temperature will eventually rise), therefore chemicals can be mobilised and excreted without causing systemic poisoning. Dr Rogers describes many case-histories in her book of patients who, for example, have severe heart disease who would certainly not tolerate a sauna, but who can tolerate FIRS very comfortably.

http://drmyhill.co.uk/wiki/Detoxing_-_Far_Infrared_Sauna_(FIRS)

Fermenting gut

The human gut is almost unique amongst mammals: the upper gut is a near-sterile, digesting, carnivorous gut (like a dog's or a cat's) to deal with meat and fat, whilst the lower gut (large bowel or colon) is full of bacteria and is a fermenting, vegetarian gut (like a horse's or cow's) to digest vegetables and fibre. From an evolutionary perspective this has been a highly successful strategy – it allows Eskimos to live on fat and protein and other people to survive on pure vegan diets.

Problems arose when humans learned to cook and to farm. This allowed them to access new foods – namely, pulses, grains and root vegetables. These need cooking to be digestible. From an evolutionary perspective this has been highly successful and allowed the population of humans to increase at a great rate. However, carbohydrates have the potential to be fermented in the upper gut with problems arising as detailed below. It is possible that some psychiatric conditions are caused by gut microbes fermenting neurotransmitters to create amphetamine- and LSD-like substances – not my idea but from a Japanese researcher called Nishihara (see References, page 122).

The stomach, duodenum and small intestine should be almost free from micro-organisms (bacteria, yeasts and parasites – that is, 'microbes'). This is normally achieved by: eating a Stone Age diet; having an acidic stomach which digests protein efficiently and kills the acid sensitive microbes; then an alkali duodenum, which kills the alkali-sensitive microbes with bicarbonate; then bile salts (which are also toxic to microbes) and pancreatic enzymes to further digest protein, fats and carbohydrates. The small intestine does more digesting and also absorbs the amino acids, fatty acids, glycerol and simple sugars that result.

Anaerobic bacteria, largely bacteroides, flourish in the large bowel, where foods that cannot be digested upstream are then fermented to produce many substances highly beneficial to the body. Bacteroides ferment soluble fibre to produce short-chain fatty acids – over 500 kCals of energy a day can be generated. This also creates heat to help keep us warm. The human body is made up of 10 trillion cells, yet in our gut we have 100 trillion microbes or more – that is, 10 times as many. Bacteria make up 60% of dry stool weight. There are over 500 different species, but 99% of microbes are from 30–40 species.

In some people there are bacteria, yeasts and possibly other parasites existing in the upper gut, which means that foods are fermented there instead of being digested. When foods get fermented this can cause symptoms and problems for many reasons such as:

- wind, bloating, heartburn and other digestive problems (so-called irritable bowel syndrome)
- malabsorption
- production of toxins through fermentation or enhanced absorption of toxic metals
- allergy to microbes in the gut (inflammatory bowel disease)
- allergy to microbes at distal sites – arthritis, interstitial cystitis, asthma, urticaria, PMR and many others
- in the longer term – cancer, diverticulitis.

http://drmyhill.co.uk/wiki/Fermentation_in_the_gut_and_CFS

Glucagon

Glucagon is the hormone that raises blood sugar levels. It does so by mobilising sugar from the liver (gluconeogenesis) and from fat stores in the body. It does the opposite to insulin. I suspect it is responsible for the symptoms of headache and nausea which often occur when people suddenly swap to low-carbohydrate, high-fat diets and the ratio between glucagon and insulin suddenly changes.

Glycogen sponge

All the products resulting from food being digested and then absorbed in the gut, pass via the portal vein to the liver. These products are toxic. So, for example, if this toxic load were to pass straight into the systemic bloodstream, then we would rapidly lose our consciousness and succumb. This occurs in liver failure. One of the toxins in the portal vein is sugar. This is like the petrol in our car – essential for it to run but highly dangerous in large amounts. The liver glycogen sponge prevents the tsunami of sugar in the portal vein from getting into the systemic bloodstream by way of a mopping-up operation. The liver achieves this by rapidly shunting sugar in the blood into the more complex storage form, glycogen, and holding it safely in the liver, from where it can be used as a pantry when blood sugar levels fall. In this respect the liver has a sponge-like effect. Should sugar levels in the systemic bloodstream fall, then the glycogen sponge can correct this by 'squeezing dry'.

Glycogen can also be stored in the muscles so these too can act as glycogen sponges to be squeezed dry, as needed.

Glycosylated/glycated haemoglobin

This is an example of an advanced glycation end product – see AGEs above (page 212). Essentially, it is a molecule where sugar has stuck on to haemoglobin. This is a metabolic mistake, but an inevitable result of the body using sugar as a fuel. It may render haemoglobin less effective. Clinically it can be used as a marker of diabetic control. The lower the level of glycosylated haemoglobin the better the control of blood sugar.

Gulf War syndrome (GWS)

GWS is the archetypal environmental illness suffered by any person involved in the Gulf Wars. It was caused by a combination of factors, including:

- Immune insult caused by many different vaccinations (up to 14 in some soldiers) given on the same day;
- Chemical warfare – organophosphate chemical weapons were used in the Gulf, notably sarin;
- Biological warfare – infectious agents were sprayed onto the troops; the organism was *Mycoplasma incognito*;
- Pyridostigmine – this is the 'antidote' to organophosphate poisoning but is toxic in its own right;
- Organophosphate pesticides, used for control of sand flies and other insects, were weekly sprayed onto tents;
- Fumes from oil-well fires;
- Uniforms were dipped in organophosphates;
- Depleted uranium resulting in radioactive exposures;

- Water from drinking and showering was often stored in tanks usually used for oil and diesel.

This was the most environmentally polluting war in history. Veterans tell me that the chemical alarms were constantly going off but the usual response was to switch the alarm off! Many of the soldiers who came back from the Gulf War with GWS are suffering, amongst other things, from a chronic infection caused by *Mycoplasma incognito*. This was developed as part of germ warfare and it may be that many thousands of the veterans are infected. Treatment is with high dose doxycycline 200 milligrams daily for six weeks, with further cycles given subsequently. To find out more about mycoplasmal infections and how to test for them, visit the website of the Institute of Molecular Medicine (http://www.immed.org/).

The symptoms of GWS are identical to those of CFS. Recently the Ministry of Defence has admitted that GWS can be caused by organophosphate poisoning. This is not at all surprising to me because the clinical features of GWS are identical to those in my 'sheep dip 'flu' farmers. By taking a careful history I often find evidence of pesticide exposure in CFS patients also – often they had not connected the chemical exposure to their symptoms. Examples include woodworm timber treatments, house fumigation, excessive use of fly sprays/Vaponas and pet flea-treatments.

This situation may not have been helped by the fact that frontline troops were told that they had to expect to function independently, without back-up, for five days, and, therefore, they had to carry with them all their needs to achieve this. Most troops chose to carry extra ammunition at the expense of carrying food. These troops were clearly carbohydrate addicts – after a few days they were not functioning normally and their bodies were perhaps more susceptible to assault from poisonings etc. After the war, the United States army commissioned a study into what would constitute the lightest but most efficient food for troops to carry. This food was found to be beta-hydroxybutyric acid; this is a ketone body produced when fats are mobilised as a fuel resource. This was produced in the form of a disgustingly flavoured drink at a dose of 1.5 grams of beta-hydroxybutyrate per kilogram of body weight per day. This drink was tested on elite athletes, who found while on it they were not hungry. All lost weight and performance increased by 7%.

http://drmyhill.co.uk/wiki/Gulf_War_Syndrome

Hypochlorhydria

Hypochlorhydria arises when the stomach becomes leaky and so cannot retain hydrochloric acid – it leaks out as fast as it is pumped in. Alternatively, the stomach becomes less efficient at producing hydrochloric acid. It is a greatly overlooked cause of problems. The stomach requires an acid environment for several reasons:

- acid is required for the digestion of protein;
- acid is required for the stomach to empty correctly, and failure to do so results in gastro-oesophageal reflux disease (and the symptom we call 'heartburn');
- acid is required to sterilise the stomach and kill microbes that may be ingested; and
- an acid environment is required for the absorption of certain micronutrients, in particular divalent and trivalent cat-ions such as calcium, magnesium, zinc, copper, iron, selenium, boron and so on.

As we age, our ability to produce stomach acid declines, but some people are simply not very good at producing stomach acid, sometimes because of pathology in the stomach (such as an allergic gastritis secondary to food intolerance), but sometimes for reasons unknown. The stomach is lined with cells that are proton pumps – that is to say they pump hydrogen ions from the bloodstream into the lumen of the stomach. Stomach acid is simply concentrated hydrogen ions.

There is a natural tendency for these hydrogen ions to diffuse back from where they came but this is prevented by very tight junctions between stomach wall cells. However, if the gut becomes inflamed for whatever reason, a 'leaky gut' (see page 234) develops and hydrogen ions leak back out. A common cause of inflammation and leaky gut is allergy.

Short-term treatment includes taking: acid supplements, such as cider vinegar; high dose ascorbic acid with meals; or betaine hydrochloride capsules. Often in the longer term, with the correct diet (low glycaemic index, low allergy potential, smaller meals), getting rid of *Helicobacter pylori*, and correcting gut flora, this cures the chronic gastritis and the stomach is again able to produce acid normally.

It is important to mitigate this extra acid with alkali. I suggest using magnesium carbonate 1 g taken 90 minutes after food, or 1-3 g last thing at night.

http://drmyhill.co.uk/wiki/Hypochlorhydria

Hypoglycaemia

'Hypoglycaemia' is the term used for blood sugar being at too low a level. To explain how this happens it is necessary to describe how sugar levels are controlled.

It is critically important for the body to maintain blood sugar levels within a narrow range. If the blood sugar level falls too low, energy supply to all tissues, particularly the brain, is impaired. However, if blood sugar levels rise too high, then this is very damaging to arteries and the long-term effect of arterial disease is heart disease and strokes. This is caused by sugar sticking to proteins and fats to make AGEs (advanced glycation end-products) which accelerate the ageing process.

Normally, the liver controls blood sugar levels. It can convert glycogen stores inside the liver to release sugar into the blood stream minute by minute in a carefully regulated way to cope with body demands, which may fluctuate from minute to minute. Excess sugar flooding into the system after a meal can be mopped up by muscles, but only so long as there is space there to act as a sponge. This occurs when we exercise as described below. This system of control works perfectly well until we upset it by eating a high carb diet and/or not exercising. Eating excessive sugar at one meal, or excessive refined carbohydrate, which is rapidly digested into sugar, can suddenly overwhelm the muscle and the liver's normal control of blood sugar levels.

We evolved over millions of years eating a diet that was very low in sugar and had no refined carbohydrate. Control of blood sugar therefore largely occurred as a result of eating this Stone Age diet and the fact that we were exercising vigorously, so any excessive sugar in the blood was quickly burned off. Nowadays the situation is different: we eat large amounts of sugar and refined carbohydrate and do not exercise sufficiently to burn off this excess sugar. The body therefore has to cope with this excessive sugar load by other mechanisms.

When food is digested, the sugars and other digestive products go straight from the gut in the portal veins to the liver, where they should all be mopped up by the liver and processed accordingly. If excessive sugar or refined carbohydrate overwhelms the liver, the sugar spills over into the systemic circulation. If not absorbed by muscle glycogen stores, high blood sugar results, which is extremely damaging to arteries. If we were exercising hard, this would be quickly burned off. However, if we are not, then other mechanisms of control are brought into play. The key player here is insulin, a hormone secreted by the pancreas. This is very good at bringing blood sugar levels down and it does so by shunting the sugar into fat. Indeed, this includes the 'bad' cholesterol LDL. There is then a rebound effect and blood sugars may well go too low – in other words, hypoglycaemia occurs. Low blood sugar is also dangerous to the body because the energy supplied to all tissues is impaired.

Subconsciously, people quickly work out that eating more sugar alleviates these symptoms, but of course they invariably overdo things; the blood sugar level then goes high and they end up on a rollercoaster ride of blood sugar level going up and down throughout the day.

Ultimately, this leads to 'metabolic syndrome' or 'syndrome X' – a major cause of disability and death in Western societies, since it is the forerunner of diabetes, obesity, cardiovascular disease, degenerative conditions and cancer.

http://drmyhill.co.uk/wiki/Hypoglycaemia_-_the_full_story

Hypothyroidism

Underactive thyroid is a very common cause of fatigue, often as a knock-on effect of a general suppression of the hypothalamic-pituitary-adrenal axis – that is, the coordinated functioning of those three glands. Symptoms of hypothyroidism arise for four reasons – either the gland itself fails (primary thyroid failure), or the pituitary gland which drives the thyroid gland into action under-functions, or there is failure to convert inactive thyroxine (T4) to its active form (T3), or there is thyroid-hormone receptor resistance. The symptoms of these four problems are the same, but blood tests show different patterns:

- In primary thyroid failure, blood tests show high levels of thyroid stimulating hormone (TSH) and low levels of T4 and T3;
- In pituitary failure, blood tests show low levels of TSH, T4 and T3;
- If there is a conversion problem, TSH and T4 may be normal, but T3 is low;
- In thyroid hormone receptor resistance there is a high TSH, high T4 and high T3.

There is another problem too, which is that the so-called

'normal range' of T4 is probably set too low. I know this because many patients with low normal T4 often improve substantially when they are started on thyroid supplements to bring levels up to the top end of the normal range.

http://drmyhill.co.uk/wiki/Hypothyroidism_-_A_Common_Hormonal_Problem_in_CFS

Inflammation

Inflammation is an essential part of our survival package. From an evolutionary perspective, the biggest killer of Homo sapiens (apart from Homo sapiens) has been infection, with cholera claiming a third of all deaths, ever. The body has to be alert to the possibility of any infection, to all of which it responds with inflammation. However, inflammation is metabolically expensive and inherently destructive. It has to be, in order to kill infections by bacteria, viruses, parasites or whatever. For example, part of the immune defence involves a 'scorched earth' policy – tissue immediately around an area of infection is destroyed so there is nothing for the invader to parasitise. The mechanism by which the immune system kills these infections is by firing free radicals at it. However, if it fires too many free radicals, then this 'friendly fire' will damage the body itself. Therefore, for inflammation to be effective it must be switched on, targeted, localised and then switched off. This entails extremely complex immune responses; clearly, there is great potential for things to go wrong.

Inflammation is also involved in the healing process. Where there is damage by trauma, there will be dead cells. Inflammation is necessary to clear away these dead cells and lay down new tissues. Inflammation is characterised by heat and redness (heat alone is antiseptic), combined with swelling, pain and loss of function, which immobilises the area being attacked by the immune system. This is necessary because physical movement will tend to massage the infection to other sites.

If one looks at life from the point of view of the immune system, it has a very difficult balancing act to manage. Too little reaction and we die from infection; too much reaction is metabolically expensive and damaging. If switched on inappropriately, the immune system has the power to kill us within seconds, an example of this being anaphylaxis.

The NO/ONOO cycle is of importance here.This is a self-perpetuating pro-inflammatory cycle described by Professor Martin Pall. It is a central part of all processes involving inflammation. I think of it as a fire which is driven by many possible factors, including poor micronutrient and anti-oxidant status, toxic stress and immune activation (infections, autoimmunity and allergy). It perpetuates many vicious cycles – for example, poor mitochondrial function results in excessive free radicals being produced which, if not mopped up by anti-oxidants, further damage and inhibit mitochondrial function.

The 'No-Oh-No' cycle (appropriately named!) seems to have a momentum of its own, and once fired up it needs all possible interventions to damp the blaze down.

http://drmyhill.co.uk/wiki/Inflammation

Inflammatory markers

If the immune system is busy in the bloodstream, then inflammatory markers are raised and can be measured. The three most commonly used are erythrocyte sedimentation rate (ESR), plasma viscosity and a C-reactive protein. Raised inflammatory markers do not tell us the cause of the inflammation, simply that something is wrong. Raised inflammatory markers should always be taken seriously and properly investigated (see my second book *Sustainable Medicine* for more detail).

Ketoacidosis

Diabetic ketoacidosis is a potentially life-threatening complication caused by a lack of insulin in the body. This may occur if the body is unable to use blood sugar (glucose) as a source of fuel.

Instead, the body breaks down fat as an alternative source of fuel. In ketosis, this breaking down of fat is desirable but because of the severity of the situation in diabetic ketoacidosis, this can lead to a dangerously high build-up of ketones.

Keto-adaptation

This is the opposite of 'metabolic inflexibility' (see page 239). It means being able to switch from burning sugar and carbs as a source of fuel to burning fat and fibre, giving the individual much longer-lasting energy and greater stamina.

Ketosis

Ketosis is a metabolic state where the majority of the body's energy supply is derived from ketone bodies in the blood. This is in contrast with a state of glycolysis where blood glucose provides the majority of the energy supply.

Leaky gut

Leaky gut means that substances which should be held in the gut leak out through the gut wall – this causes many problems:

- Hydrogen ions (ie acid) cannot be concentrated in the stomach, leading to hypochlorhydria (see page 228). This causes malabsorption of minerals and vitamin B12. Hypochlorhydria is a major risk factor for fermenting gut since acid helps to sterilise the upper gut. It also is an essential part of protein digestion.
- Allergy – Normally one expects foods to be completely broken down into amino acids (from protein), essential fatty acids and glycerol (from fats) and single sugars, or 'monosaccharides' (from carbohydrates). The undigested foods stay in the gut and the small digested molecules pass through the gut wall into the portal bloodstream and on to the liver where they are dealt with. However, leaky gut means food particles get absorbed before they have been

properly digested. This means large food molecules get into the bloodstream. These large molecules are 'interesting' to the immune system, which may mistake them for viruses and/or bacteria. In this event, it may attack these harmless molecules, either with antibodies or directly with immune cells. This causes inflammation. Inflammation in the gut causes diseases of the gut. Inflammation elsewhere can cause almost any symptom you care to mention. It may switch on allergy and/or auto-immunity – that is, it is potentially a disease-amplifying process.

- Another problem with small digested molecules or polypeptides getting in to the bloodstream is that these molecules may be biologically active. Some of them act as hormone mimics, which can affect levels of glucose in the blood or blood pressure. This is akin to throwing a handful of sand into a finely tuned machine – it makes a real mess of homeostatic (balancing) mechanisms of controlling body activities.

http://drmyhill.co.uk/wiki/Leaky_gut_syndrome

Lipids, fats and essential fatty acids

The vast majority of cell metabolism takes place on, in or around cell membranes. The structure of cell membranes is identical throughout the animal kingdom. They are made up of fatty molecules which have a water-loving end and a fat-loving end; these combine in a sandwich so the fat-loving end forms the core of the membrane and the water-loving end the outside of the membrane. The structure of the membrane and how liquid it is depends on the fats that are in it. If the composition of membranes changes, then they will either become more stiff or more liquid.

There are a great many effects which result from this, for example increased irritability and sensitivity, which of course could explain many CFS symptoms, such as intolerance of chemicals and foods, intolerance of heat, light and touch, low pain threshold, cardiac dysarrhythmias and so on. Indeed, a great many drugs work because of their effects on changing membrane structure, such as general anaesthetics, tranquilisers, pain killers and anti-inflammatory drugs.

Mitochondrial membranes are different from cell membranes because they have to be a little stiffer in order to hold still the bundles of enzymes called cristae on which oxidative phosphorylation takes place. They have an additional fat – namely 'cardiolipin' – to create this extra stiffness.

Having the correct oils in the diet are essential for energy supply to the brain. Poor energy supply means foggy brain.

http://drmyhill.co.uk/wiki/Lipids,_fats_and_essential_fatty_acids

Lipodystrophy

'Lipodystrophy' simply means that fat is not laid down in a uniform way – it looks and feels lumpy. This often occurs, for example, at the site of repeated injections. Cellulite is a form of lypodystrophy which, I suspect, is also related to metabolic syndrome. Cellulite, or the prevention of such, can be a useful lever for persuading the young and vain to do a low-carb diet.

Magnesium

Magnesium is an essential mineral required for at least 300 different enzyme systems in the body. It is centrally involved in the energy delivery systems of the body, ie the mitochondria.

Red blood cell levels of magnesium are almost invariably low in patients with CFS. Furthermore, very many patients with CFS benefit from magnesium by injection.

I believe that a low red cell magnesium is a symptom of mitochondrial failure. It is the job of mitochondria to produce ATP for cell metabolism and about 40% of all mitochondrial output goes into maintaining calcium/magnesium and sodium/potassium ion pumps. I suspect that when mitochondria fail, these pumps malfunction and therefore calcium leaks into cells and magnesium leaks out. This, of course, compounds the underlying mitochondrial failure because calcium is toxic to mitochondria and magnesium necessary for normal mitochondrial function. This is just one of the many vicious cycles we see in patients with fatigue syndromes. The reason for giving magnesium by injection is in order to reduce the work of the calcium/magnesium ion pump by reducing the concentration gradient across cell membranes.

http://www.drmyhill.co.uk/wiki/Magnesium

Malabsorption

The job of the gut is to absorb the goodness from food. To do this, it first has to reduce food particles to a size which allows the digestive enzymes to get at them; then it has to provide the correct acidity then alkalinity for enzymes to work, produce the necessary enzymes and emulsifying agent (bile salts), and move the food along the gut. Finally, the large bowel allows growth of bacteria for a final digestive/fermentative process and water extraction. The gut has a particularly difficult job because it has to identify foods that are safe from potentially dangerous microbes (most are not dangerous but positively beneficial). This explains why 90% of the immune system is gut associated. The innoculation of the gut with these gut-friendly microbes takes place in the first few minutes following birth.

Anything which goes wrong with any of these processes can cause malabsorption. Malabsorption means that the body does not get the raw materials for normal everyday work and repair. Consequently, there is the potential for much to go wrong.

http://drmyhill.co.uk/wiki/Malabsorption_-_failure_to_get_the_goodness_from_food

Mercury poisoning

The early symptoms of mercury poisoning can be variable

but may include loss of short-term memory, a metallic taste in the mouth (this is difficult since taste is relative and dental amalgam is constantly present) and fine tremor. Mercury may also cause personality changes (like the Mad Hatter from *Alice in Wonderland*, which was written at a time when hatters used mercury in hat-making). It is also toxic to the nerves of the heart and may be a cause of electrical dysrhythmias (palpitations).

Dental amalgam is the commonest source of mercury poisoning. Professor Fritz Lorscheider's work over many years has looked at how mercury leaches out from dental amalgam. At room temperature, mercury is a liquid and in dental amalgam it is not chemically bound into the amalgam, but there as a liquid, albeit a very tough and stiff liquid. He took sheep, filled their molars with dental amalgam which was radioactively labelled and four months later scanned the sheep to see if the mercury had migrated; he discovered that it had deposited in their hearts, bones, kidneys and brains. He then looked at what mercury does in the brain. He found that at concentrations lower than those present in the saliva of a person with amalgam fillings, nerve fibres collapsed because they could not build their essential structure. (For more detail see the link below.)

The pathology he found is similar to Alzheimer's disease, in which neuro-fibrillary tangles are formed. Essentially, Lorscheider's findings tell us that mercury causes Alzheimer's disease. Alzheimer's is also associated with aluminium poisoning and, indeed, aluminium is a very similar metal to mercury in the periodic table of elements. The main source of aluminium is from antacids, antiperspirants and cooking foil, pots and pans.

In California, Sweden and Germany mercury amalgam has been banned. Recently it has been banned in Norway.

http://drmyhill.co.uk/wiki/Mercury_Toxicity_of_Dental_Amalgam_Why_you_should_have_your_dental_amalgams_removed

Metabolic inflexibility

Metabolic inflexibility is the condition that arises when the body cannot switch from burning sugars and starches as its fuel source to running on fibres and fats. This is the opposite of keto-adaptation – that is, the metabolic condition which arises when the body is powering itself from fat and ketones.

Metabolic syndrome

This is the clinical picture which arises when the body powers itself predominantly with sugars and carbohydrates. There is a loss of control over blood sugar levels. The conventional definition of metabolic syndrome only occurs in an advanced state of such – that is, when there is a combination of abdominal (central) obesity (i.e. being apple shaped), high blood pressure, high fasting sugar, high triglycerides and low levels of friendly high density lipoprotein (HDL). My advice is not to wait for these nasty and damaging features to emerge, but to tackle the metabolic syndrome early.

Micronutrients

Micronutrients are substances required in trace amounts for the normal growth and development of living organisms. While these should all be adequately supplied by our diet, the problem is that modern Western diets do not deliver. As a supplement I recommend that everyone take a basic package of supplements, which includes a multivitamin supplement, multiminerals, essential fatty acids (omega-6 and -3 in the proportion of 4:1, such as one tablespoon of hemp oil) with additional vitamins D, B12 and C.

A good multivitamin is easy to purchase. However, I have been unable to find a good multimineral preparation which contains all essential minerals in adequate amounts, in the correct proportion and in a form which is is soluble and easily absorbed. So I formulated my own product which has in addition extra vitamin B12 and vitamin D. This physiological Multi Mineral Mix (MMM) is not to be confused with 'Miracle Mineral Solution' (MMS), about which the Food Standards Agency has issued an urgent warning. My MMM is a mix of minerals which you make up in water that are all essential for human metabolism. The amounts given below are elemental weights of the pure mineral. These amounts are those considered desirable from modern nutrition research and are mostly above the 'recommended daily amount' (RDA). These RDA amounts were set down in 1941 and are now outdated. If better preparations become available or I learn more about essential minerals, then the composition of MMM may change. The newest formulation contains B12 1 milligram per gram (mg/g) of MMM and vitamin D, 1000 iu (international units) per gram.

- Calcium (as calcium chloride) – 60 mg
- Magnesium (as magnesium chloride) – 70 mg
- Potassium (as potassium chloride) – 40 mg
- Zinc (as zinc chloride) – 6 mg
- Iron (as ferric ammonium chloride) – 3 mg
- Boron (as sodium borate) – 2 mg
- Iodine (as potassium iodate) – 0.3 mg
- Copper (as copper sulphate) – 0.2 mg
- Manganese (as manganese chloride) – 0.2 mg
- Molybdenum (as sodium molybdate) – 40 mcg
- Selenium (as sodium selenate) – 40 mcg
- Chromium (as chromium chloride) – 40 mcg
- Vitamin B12 – 1000 mcg/g
- Vitamin D (as cholecalciferol) – 1000 iu

Dosage: the daily dose of MMM is one gram (one blue scoop) per two stone (12.5 kilograms) of body weight to a maximum of 5 grams (five scoops) per day. This dose assumes that you get nothing from food. However, as your diet improves and deficiencies are corrected the dose can be reduced – most people need just 2-3 grams daily for maintenance of good health.

The daily dose should be dissolved in cold water – half a pint of water per 1 gram of the mix (the maximum dose made up in three pints of water) and taken throughout the day. You should start off with just half a pint of mix daily and build up slowly to allow your stomach to adjust to the changes; otherwise it may cause nausea and loose bowel movements. Ideally, use with ascorbic acid (vitamin C) to optimise absorption. The juice of half a lemon makes this more palatable. It also makes one drink water; this is something many people forget to do. MMM is suitable for all age groups, including babies and pregnant women. The dose is not critical as there is a wide margin of safety for all essential minerals. The mix is 100% active ingredient with no additives, colourings, flavourings or bulking substances. The formula is completely stable and will last for many years. Keep the lid tightly screwed on to the jar; otherwise moisture from the air may be absorbed and the minerals change colour. This does not matter, but the contents may go hard or discolour slightly.

Vitamin C can be taken with the MMMs and/or at night. The idea here is that vitamin C helps to keep microbes in the upper gut at a low level (you can never completely sterilise the upper gut). Vitamin C kills all microbes, including viruses.

http://drmyhill.co.uk/wiki/Nutritional_Supplements__what_everybody_should_be_taking_all_the_time_even_if_nothing_is_wrong

Minerals

You could argue that we all die ultimately from mineral and vitamin deficiencies. People who traditionally live to a great age are often found living in areas watered by streams from glaciers. Glaciers are lakes of ice which have spent the previous few thousand years crunching up rocks. Therefore the waters coming from the glaciers are rich in minerals. This is used not just to drink but to irrigate crops and to bathe in. These people therefore have had excellent levels of micronutrients throughout life. Given the right raw materials, things do not go wrong in the body and ageing is slowed. For example:

- Low magnesium and selenium is a risk factor for heart disease
- Low selenium increases risk of cancer
- Copper is necessary to make elastic tissue – deficiency causes weaknesses in arteries leading to aneurysms
- Low chromium increases the risk of diabetes
- Good antioxidant status (vitamins A, C, E and selenium) slows the ageing process
- Superoxide dismutase enzymes require zinc, copper and manganese to function
- Iodine is necessary to make thyroid hormones and is highly protective against breast disease
- The immune system needs a huge range of minerals to work well, especially zinc, selenium and magnesium
- Boron is highly protective against arthritis
- Magnesium is required in at least 300 enzyme systems
- Zinc is needed for normal brain development; a deficiency at a critical stage of development causes dyslexia
- Any deficiency of selenium, zinc, copper or magnesium can cause infertility
- Iron prevents anaemia
- Molybdenum is necessary to detox sulphites.

The secret of success is to copy Nature. Civilisation and Western diets have brought great advantages, but at the same time are responsible for escalating death rates from cancer, heart disease and dementia. I want the best of both worlds. I like my warm kitchen, fridge, wood-burning cooker, computer and telly, but I want to eat and live in the environment in which primitive man thrived.

http://drmyhill.co.uk/wiki/Minerals

MMM

This is my 'multi-mineral mix' that I formulated in the absence of any product that delivered the optimum combination of supplementary minerals I recommend. See 'Micronutrients', page 239, for more details.

NAD – nicotinamide adenine dinucleotide, niacinamide and nicotinic amide

Nicotinamide is vitamin B3, vital to make NAD which is an essential part of energy delivery mechanisms within mitochondria. Though present in meat, eggs and whole grains, it is such a common deficiency that we should all be taking a supplement (at least 500 mg daily, possibly 1500 mg slow release) to slow the ageing process.

Neutralisation

Neutralisation is a technique to turn off allergies. A small amount of antigen (food, inhalant or chemical) is injected into the skin to elicit a skin reaction and possibly symptoms. The injection is repeated at progressively greater dilutions until the 'neutralising' dose is found, at which level there is no skin reaction and symptoms are switched off. The patient then self-treats daily with this neutralising dose, possibly with drops under the tongue or injections. It is a laborious technique since every antigen has to be neutralised to individually – furthermore the neutralisation end points can change. However, it is helpful to identify allergies where there is uncertainty.

Nickel

Nickel (Ni) is a nasty toxic metal and a known carcinogen. It is one of the metals we see most commonly in toxicity tests – it appears stuck onto DNA, stuck on to translocator protein and is often present in blood at high levels. Nickel is a problem because biochemically it 'looks' like zinc. Zinc deficiency is very common in people eating Western diets, so if the body needs zinc and it is not there, it will use look-alike nickel instead. But nickel does not do the job and, indeed, gets in the way of normal biochemistry. Zinc is an essential co-factor in many enzyme systems from alcohol dehydrogenase to zinc carboxypeptidase, so there is enormous potential for harm from nickel. Nickel sensitivity is very common and often diagnosed from rashes from jewellery, zips, watches etc. What we know from people with chemical sensitivity is that they often have toxic loads of those things they are sensitive to. So nickel sensitivity often equates with nickel toxicity.

Nickel is unavoidable if you live a Western lifestyle. Many industrial processes release nickel into the atmosphere.

- Stainless steel contains 14 per cent nickel; this includes cookware and eating utensils. Use cast iron pans, glass or ceramic.
- Jewellery – used because it is such a versatile, malleable metal. Well absorbed with piercing.
- Catalytic converters in cars release fine particulate nickel into the atmosphere – so fine that it cannot be filtered out by the lining of the bronchus, so it is well absorbed by inhalation and easily gets into blood vessels. Here it triggers inflammation and arterial disease.
- Cigarette smoke.
- Medical prostheses.

http://drmyhill.co.uk/wiki/Nickel_-_a_nasty_toxic_metal

Nutritional supplements

See Micronutrients.

http://drmyhill.co.uk/wiki/Nutritional_Supplements_what_everybody_should_be_taking_all_the_time_even_if_nothing_is_wrong

Organophosphate (OP) poisoning

This is a remarkably common but under-diagnosed problem because we are all constantly exposed to organophosphates, including glyphosate – this (Round-up is the best known product) is generally regarded as safe, but this is not so.

Different people have different symptoms of OP poisoning. Symptoms depend partly on how much OP they have been exposed to, whether they have had single massive exposure, or chronic sub-lethal exposure, whether it has been combined with other chemicals, and how good their body is at coping with toxic chemicals. Symptoms divide into the following categories:

No obvious symptoms at all – A government-sponsored study at the Institute of Occupational Medicine that looked at farmers who regularly handled OPs but who were complaining of no symptoms, showed that they suffered from mild brain damage. Their ability to think clearly and problem solve was impaired.

Sheep dip 'flu (mild acute poisoning) – This is a 'flu-like illness which follows exposure to OPs. Sometimes the farmer just has a bit of a headache, feels unusually tired or finds he can't think clearly. This may just last a few hours to a few days and the sufferer recovers completely. Most sufferers do not realise that they have been poisoned and put any symptoms down to a hard day's work. It can occur after dipping, but some farmers will get symptoms after the slightest exposure, such as visiting markets and inhaling OP fumes from fleeces.

Acute organophosphate poisoning – This is the syndrome recognised by doctors and Poisons Units. Symptoms occur within 24 hours of exposure and include collapse, breathing problems, sweating, diarrhoea, vomiting, excessive salivation, heart dysrhythmias, extreme anxiety etc. Treatment is with atropine. You have to have a large dose of OP to have this effect (such as, drink some of the dip!) and so this syndrome is rarely seen.

Intermediate syndrome – This occurs 1-3 weeks after exposure and is characterised by weakness of shoulder, neck and upper leg muscles. It is rarely diagnosed because it goes unrecognised.

Long-term chronic effects – These symptoms develop in some susceptible individuals. They can either occur following a single massive exposure, or after several years of regular sub-lethal exposure to OPs. Essentially there is an acceleration of the normal ageing process with arterial disease, heart disease, cancer and dementia presenting at a young age.

The treatment follows the same principles as for any chemical poisoning (see Chemical poisoning, page 218).

Fortunately, most farmers are intelligent and realise the above state of affairs, but the lack of street credibility and help from government agencies make this illness a social and financial disaster area.

http://drmyhill.co.uk/wiki/Organophosphate_Poisoning_-_symptoms_and_treatment

Osteoporosis

Osteoporosis is a modern disease of Western society. Primitive societies eating Stone Age diets do not suffer from osteoporosis. So the underlying principle for avoiding osteoporosis is that we should mimic primitive cultures eating a Stone Age diet and living a toxin free life. This does not mean you need to run around half naked in a rabbit-skin loin cloth depriving yourself of the pleasures of 21st-century Western life. We need to cherry pick from the good things of all civilisations.

To make good quality bone you need the raw materials (Stone Age diet and supplements), the ability to absorb minerals (an acid stomach), the drive to lay these down in bone (exercise, vitamin D, DHEA) and an alkali body to prevent minerals being washed out in urine (magnesium carbonate at night). I have collected before and after bone density scans of 14 patients doing these regimes. In all cases, the bone density has remained the same or increased. So whilst the numbers are small the statistics are powerful.

Dairy products and calcium supplements alone make osteoporosis worse. This is because calcium in isolation blocks the absorption of other essential minerals, such as magnesium. Vitamin D is the key to calcium – it promotes the absorption of calcium (and magnesium) and ensures its deposition in bone.

The medical profession would have us believe that the only important constituent of bone is calcium. Actually bone is made up of many different minerals, including magnesium, calcium, potassium, boron, silicon, manganese, iron, zinc, copper, chromium, strontium and maybe others. For its formation it also requires a whole range of vitamins, essential fatty acids and amino acids.

http://www.drmyhill.co.uk/wiki/Osteoporosis_-_practical_nutritional_considerations

Pain

Although pain seems like 'a pain', actually it is essential for our survival. Pain protects us from ourselves. It prevents us from damaging our bodies. Indeed, people who are born with no pain perception look as if they have been traumatised – they are covered in cuts, bruises and sores, because they are unaware that they are damaging themselves. Pain is the local method of avoiding damage – it makes us protect the affected part of the body and makes us keep it still so that healing and repair can take place. If pain becomes more generalised then pain is accompanied by fatigue. What this means is that chronic pain and chronic fatigue go hand in hand and therefore so should treatment. We learn through experience what is painful; this makes us avoid those painful experiences and therefore protects our bodies.

Although it is desirable to learn about pain, this can also cause problems because if the underlying causes of the pain are not identified we 'learn' more pain. In the ideal situation, we damage our bodies with say a cut or bruise and the local pain makes us care for that damaged area by protecting it and keeping it still so that healing and repair can take place. With healing the pain goes. If the root source of the pain is not identified, it creates a problem because then the pain increases. The body naturally thinks that increasing pain means we will take more care, identify the source of the pain, keep the limb more still and therefore the body winds up the pain signal to try to elicit the appropriate response. Effectively we learn to feel more pain because there is an upgrading of this pain response. This is not a psychological effect – this actually occurs within the cells themselves. This makes it very important to identify causes of pain early on in any disease process and allow time for healing and repair, otherwise the pain will get worse.

http://drmyhill.co.uk/wiki/Pain

Pancreatic function

The pancreas is a large gland which lies behind the stomach and upper gut. It has two major functions of clinical importance. Firstly, it acts as an endocrine organ to produce insulin and other hormones essential for the control of blood sugar. Secondly, it has an exocrine function to produce enzymes essential for the digestion of food. These enzymes include those to digest proteins, fats and starches and to work best they need an alkali environment. When food is present in the duodenum and jejunum, the gall bladder contracts, sending a bolus of bile salts which combines with bicarbonate and pancreatic enzymes to allow digestion to take place in the duodenum and jejunum.

If the pancreas does not produce sufficient digestive enzymes and bicarbonate, then foods will not be digested. This can lead to problems downstream. Firstly, foods may be fermented instead of being digested and this can produce the symptom of bloating due to wind, together with metabolites such as various alcohols, hydrogen sulphide and other toxic compounds. Secondly, foods are not fully broken down so that they cannot be absorbed and this can result in malabsorption.

Where there is severe pancreatic dysfunction it is obvious because the stools themselves become greasy and fatty, foul smelling, bulky and difficult to flush away. Where there is malabsorption of fat, there will be malabsorption of essential fatty acids such as the omega-3 and omega-6 fatty acids, and there will be malabsorption of fat-soluble vitamins such as vitamins A, D, E and K. If foods are poorly digested, this results in large antigenically interesting molecules appearing downstream, which alerts the immune system and could switch on allergies – that is, poor digestion of food is a risk factor for allergy.

Where there is poor pancreatic function digestive aids can be very helpful. I use pancreatic enzymes together with magnesium carbonate 90 minutes after food (not with food since we need a 90-minute window of time of acidity for stomach function). High-dose pancreatic enzymes have revolutionised the treatment of cystic fibrosis.

http://drmyhill.co.uk/wiki/Pancreatic_exocrine_function

Prion disorders

I think of prion disorders as protein cancers. Prions are proteins which are normally present in the body and perform essential functions. However, if they come into contact with a particular toxin or heavy metal or another twisted prion (rotten apple effect), then they too twist and distort. When they twist in such a way that they cannot be broken down by the body's enzyme systems, they cause problems because the body has to dump them as it cannot break them down. Pathologically this is known as amyloid. This results in deposition of these indigestible proteins and this can occur anywhere in the body.

Cancers, of course, are simply cells which replicate themselves and build up to cause problems. Viruses are strips of DNA which replicate themselves and build up in the body to cause problems. Difficulties arise when they literally get in the way of the body and stop it functioning normally. Although amyloid can occur anywhere in the body, the biggest problem is in the brain, perhaps partly because it is a closed box and therefore there is not any room for all this excess protein to be dumped and partly because each part of the brain is unique and any loss of function is quickly noticed. So these protein cancers tend to cause problems which may take many years to develop and so far the medical profession has no method of slowing down this process. The conditions they cause include Alzheimer's disease; Parkinson's disease; Creutzfeldt-Jacob's disease; motor neurone disease; and multisystem atrophy (MSA). We are currently seeing an epidemic of these conditions – the number of people suffering from them is increasing fast. Not my words but the words of Professor Colin Pritchard, professor of epidemiological medicine at Southampton University. They are an inevitable part of Western lifestyles and diets high in sugar and refined carbohydrate. Indeed, Alzheimer's has been dubbed type 3 diabetes of the brain.

http://www.drmyhill.co.uk/wiki/Prion_disorders

Probiotics

In a normal situation free from antiseptics, antibiotics, high-carbohydrate diets, bottle feeding, hormones and other such accoutrements of modern western life, the gut flora is safe. Babies start life in mother's womb with a sterile gut (although interestingly there is some evidence that their gut becomes innoculated before birth through transfer of microbes across the placenta!). During the process of birth, they become inoculated with bacteria from the birth canal and perineum. These bacteria are largely bacteroides which cannot survive for more than a few minutes outside the human gut. This inoculation is enhanced through breast-feeding because the first milk, namely colostrum, is highly desirable substrate for these bacteria to flourish. We now know that this is an essential part of immune programming. Indeed, 90% of the immune system is gut associated. These essential probiotics programme the immune system so that they accept them and learn what is beneficial. A healthy gut flora therefore is highly protective against invasion of the gut by other strains of bacteria or viruses. The problem is there is no probiotic on the market that supplies bacteroides, for the above reasons. If we eat probiotics which have been artificially cultured, for a short while the levels of these probiotics in the gut do increase. However, as soon as we stop eating them, levels taper off and may disappear. Ideally for bacteria to be accepted into the normal gut and remain, they have to be programmed first through somebody else's gut (in this case, mother's).

So, when it comes to repleting gut flora, there are two ways that we can go about this – either we can take probiotics very regularly (and the cheapest way to do this is to grow your own probiotics) or to take bacteroides directly. Indeed, this latter technique is well established in the treatment of *Clostridium difficile* (a normally fatal gastroenteritis in humans) and interestingly in idiopathic diarrhoea in horses. In the latter case horses are inoculated with the bacteria from the gut of another horse. These ideas have been developed further by Dr Thomas Borody with his ideas on faecal bacteriotherapy, which can provide a permanent cure in cases of ulcerative colitis, severe constipation, *clostridium difficile* infections and pseudomembranous colitis. The reason this technique works so well is because the most abundant bacteria in the large bowel, bacteroides, cannot survive outside the human gut and cannot be given by any other route.

The gut flora is extremely stable and difficult to change. Therefore if you are going to take probiotics, you have to be prepared to take them for the long term. Many preparations on the market are ineffective. Those found to be most effective are those milk ferments and live yoghurts where the product is freshly made. It is not really surprising. Keeping bacteria alive is difficult and it is not surprising that they do not survive dehydration and storage at room temperature.

So your best chance of eating live viable bacteria is to buy live yoghurts or drinks. These can be easily grown at home, just as one would make home-made yoghurt. If you cannot grow easily from a culture, then it suggests that the culture is not active, so this is a good test of what is and is not viable. I have tried to culture on soya and coconut milks from dried extracts with very poor success rates, suggesting that the dried extracts are not viable in the gut.

The use of probiotics is already established practice in animal welfare and probiotics are actively marketed to the horse industry for this very reason. Furthermore, probiotics are routinely used in the pig industry to prevent post-weaning diarrhoea. Anyone who has to take antibiotics for any reason should take these cultures as a routine to prevent 'super-infection' with undesirable bugs. These cultures are also an essential part of re-colonising the gut following gut eradication therapy.

http://drmyhill.co.uk/wiki/Probiotics_we_should_all_be_taking_these_all_the_time_and_double_the_dose_following_antibiotics_and_gastroenteritis

Sleep

Humans evolved to sleep when it is dark and wake when it is light. Sleep is a form of hibernation when the body shuts down in order to repair damage done through use, to conserve energy and to hide from predators. The normal sleep pattern that evolved in hot climates is to sleep, keep warm and conserve energy during the cold nights and then to sleep again in the afternoons when it is too hot to work and to hide away from the midday sun. As humans migrated away from the Equator, the sleep pattern had to change with the seasons and as the lengths of the days changed.

After the First World War a strain of Spanish 'flu swept

through Europe killing 50 million people worldwide. Some people sustained neurological damage and for some this virus wiped out their sleep centre in the brain. This meant they were unable to sleep at all. All these unfortunate people were dead within two weeks and this was the first solid scientific evidence that sleep was as essential for life as food and water. Indeed, all living creatures require a regular 'sleep' (or period of quiescence) during which time healing and repair take place. You must put as much work into your sleep as your diet. Without a good night's sleep on a regular basis all other interventions are undermined.

http://drmyhill.co.uk/wiki/Sleep_is_vital_for_good_health_-_especially_in_CFS

Stone Age diet

Human beings evolved over millions of years eating particular foods. Neanderthal man was a carnivore and only ever ate meat, fish and shell fish. Fat would have been a treasured food. The carbohydrate content would have been, for much of the year, zero. More recently Paleolithic man expanded the diet to include root vegetables, fruits, nuts and seeds which he could scavenge from the wild, but even these would only be available occasionally in season. It is only in the last few thousand years since the Persians, Egyptians and Romans that we began farming, and grains and dairy products were introduced into the human diet. A few thousand years from an evolutionary point of view is almost negligible. Many people have simply failed to adapt to cope with carbohydrates and dairy products and it is very likely that these foods cause a range of health problems in susceptible people.

Modern studies on ancient tribes who continue to eat a Stone Age (Paleolithic) diet show that these people do not suffer from diabetes, obesity, heart disease or cancer. If they can survive the ravages of the cold, infectious diseases, childbirth and war wounds, then these people live healthily to a great age. I am coming to the view that whatever our medical problem may be, or even if we simply want to stay well, we should all move towards eating a Stone Age diet based on protein (meat, fish, eggs), fat and vegetable fibre. Recent Western diets get 70% of their calories from wheat, dairy products, sugar and potato and it is no surprise that these are the major causes of modern ill health such as cancer, heart disease, diabetes, obesity and degenerative disorders. Traditional Chinese diets have no dairy products, no gluten grains, no alcohol and no fruit.

http://drmyhill.co.uk/wiki/Stone_Age_Diet_-_this_is_a_diet_which_we_all_should_follow

Syndrome X

This is another name for the pre-diabetic state called 'metabolic syndrome' in this book, when blood sugar levels see-saw between too high and too low. See Hyoglycaemia, page 229.

http://drmyhill.co.uk/wiki/Hypoglycaemia_-_the_full_story

Toxins

These are substances that are dangerous to the body because they inhibit normal metabolism, damage the structure of the body or are wasteful of its resources. Organophosphates, for example, inhibit oxidative phosphorylation. Toxic metals can stick onto DNA and trigger cancer; they also stick on to proteins to trigger prion disorders. Products of the fermenting gut require energy and micronutrients for the liver to deal with them. Volatile organic compounds may need methylating to detoxify them and this is a drain on folic acid and vitamin B12.

Toxins come from the outside world (exogenous) and the inside world (endogenous). Exogenous toxins include POPs (persistent organic pollutants), metals, radiation (most of this comes from the medical profession), toxic halides (fluorides, bromides) and many more. A major source of toxic stress is from prescription medication. Endogenous toxins come from the fermenting gut, natural toxins in foods (e.g. lectins, mycotoxins), breakdown products of normal metabolism, from inflammation, and other such.

Modern Western lifestyles mean we are inevitably exposed to chemicals. See my website for a checklist of exogenous toxins and their sources.

http://drmyhill.co.uk/wiki/Chemical_poisons_and_toxins

Transdermal micronutrients

I see many patients for whom we know what the micronutrient deficiency is that causes their problem, but giving those micronutrients by mouth does not help, or indeed makes them worse. What I suspect is getting in the way is the gut. For micronutrients to get into the body to do good they must first get there! To achieve this we need the ability to digest and absorb them and the energy to do this. I suspect the latter is a problem for many of my severe CFS patients. Food allergy, the fermenting gut and poor stomach, liver and pancreatic function may all be problems. This may explain why so many of my sick patients do well on injections of micronutrients.

To get round this problem I use transdermal preparations to be sprayed onto the skin. A key ingredient is DMSO – this passes through skin like a knife through butter and carries through everything dissolved within it. DMSO is a naturally occurring organic sulphur-containing molecule, derived from tree bark and closely related to MSM (a useful treatment for arthritis). The early clinical feedback has been encouraging – but watch this space!

Transdermal magnesium seems to be especially effective in muscle, joint, tendon and connective tissue problems. I suspect the mechanism of this is that magnesium reduces the friction within tissues.

http://drmyhill.co.uk/wiki/Transdermal_micronutrients

Vitamin D and sunshine

Western cultures have become almost phobic about any exposure of unprotected skin to sunshine. This phobia is based on the perceived risk of skin cancers. However, the two skin cancers which are known to because by sunshine, namely basal and squamous cell cancers, are easily diagnosed and treated – people very rarely die from these tumours.

The most serious skin cancer is melanoma. This does not appear most commonly on sun-exposed skin. Schools of thought now believe melanoma is not caused by sunshine. Indeed, sunshine is highly protective against all cancers – the key is to tan but not burn. In efforts to avoid burning, the US Environmental Protection Agency is currently advising that ultraviolet light, and therefore sunlight, is so dangerous that we should 'protect ourselves against ultraviolet light whenever we can see our shadow'. This is a nonsense.

Sun exposure is essential for normal good health in order to produce vitamin D – and partly as a result of current recommendations, we are seeing declining levels of vitamin D. There is an interesting inverse correlation between sunshine exposure, vitamin D levels, and incidence of disease as one moves away from the Equator. Even correcting for other factors, such as diet, there is strong evidence to show that vitamin D protects against osteoarthritis, osteoporosis, bone fractures (vitamin D strengthens the muscles thereby improving balance and movement and preventing falls), cancer, hypertension, hypercholesterolaemia, diabetes, heart disease, multiple sclerosis and vulnerability to infections. Multiple sclerosis is a particularly interesting example of a possible vitamin D deficiency disease. Indeed, mice bred for susceptibility to multiple sclerosis can be completely protected against development of this disease by feeding them high doses of vitamin D.

Human beings evolved over hundreds of thousands of years in equatorial areas and were daily exposed to sunshine. Dark skins evolved to protect against sun damage. However, as hominids migrated north, those races which retained their dark skins were unable to make sufficient vitamin D in the skin and did not survive. Only those hominids with paler skins survived. Thus the further away from the Equator, the paler the skin became. Races in polar areas survived because they were able to get an alternative source of vitamin D from fish and seafood.

http://drmyhill.co.uk/wiki/Vitamin_D_and_Sunshine:_an_essential_vitamin!_Protects_against_cancer,_heart_and_bone_disease

Yeast problems and candida

Yeast is one of the common fermenting microbes in the upper gut and is part of the upper fermenting gut issue (see above). Yeast problems are an inevitable problem of Western diets, which are high in carbohydrates. The problem is worsened by antibiotics, the Pill and HRT.

Problems may arise initially because yeast numbers build up, sometimes to produce overt infections such as oral thrush, perineal thrush or skin tinea infections (ringworm, athlete's foot, fungal toenails, tinea etc). With chronic exposures there is the potential to sensitise to yeast and that causes much worse problems, characterised by itching, pain and inflammation. Psoriasis may be allergy to yeast; ditto chronic cystitis and interstitial cystitis.

Index

Also by Dr Sarah Myhill

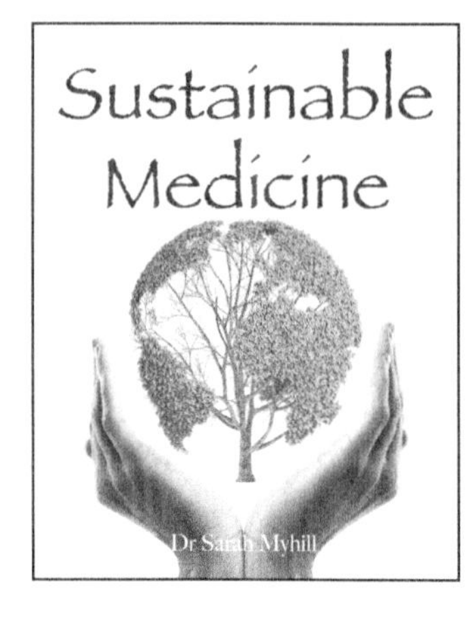

The starting point for treating all symptoms and diseases. Sustainable Medicine explains why we have symptoms and details how we can work out their causes, appropriate tests and the tools to effect a cure.

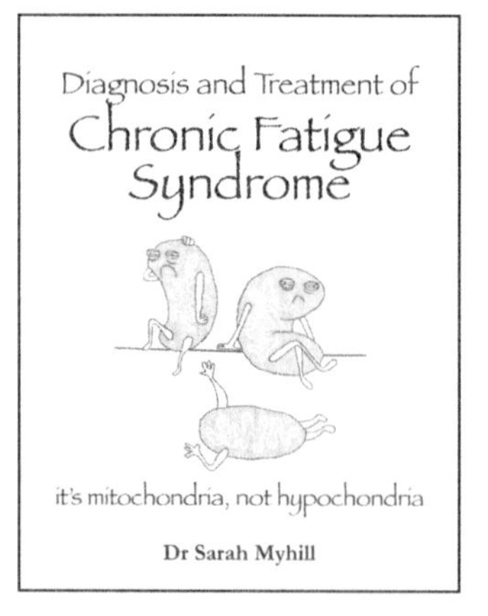

Dr Myhill explores the commonest symptom that people take to their doctor - fatigue - and its pathological end result if the symptom is ignored.

www.hammersmithbooks.co.uk

The PK Cookbook

Go Paleo-Ketogenic and Get the Best of Both Worlds

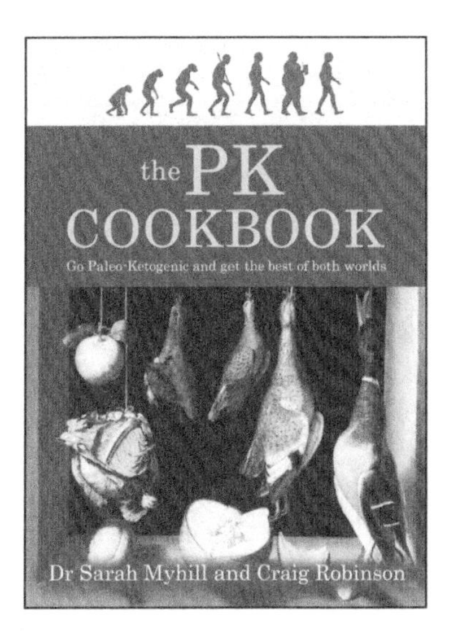

Prevent & Cure Diabetes has given you the intellectual imperatives - the 'why' - to adopt a paleo-ketogenic diet. *The PK Cookbook* gives you the 'how'. Based on Dr Myhill's firsthand experience of adopting this diet herself and guiding her patients through implementing it, she has found that the 'PK bread' has helped more people stick to this healthy way of eating than any other recipe.